T0296679

LANDSCAPES OF ACTIVISM

Medical Anthropology: Health, Inequality, and Social Justice

Series editor: Lenore Manderson

Books in the Medical Anthropology series are concerned with social patterns of and social responses to ill health, disease, and suffering, and how social exclusion and social justice shape health and healing outcomes. The series is designed to reflect the diversity of contemporary medical anthropological research and writing and will offer scholars a forum to publish work that showcases the theoretical sophistication, methodological soundness, and ethnographic richness of the field.

Books in the series may include studies on the organization and movement of peoples, technologies, and treatments; how inequalities pattern access to these; and how individuals, communities, and states respond to various assaults on well-being, including from illness, disaster, and violence.

Carina Heckert, *Fault Lines of Care: Gender, HIV, and Global Health in Bolivia*
Joel Christian Reed, *Landscapes of Activism: Civil Society and HIV and AIDS Care in Northern Mozambique*

LANDSCAPES OF ACTIVISM

Civil Society and HIV and AIDS Care in Northern Mozambique

JOEL CHRISTIAN REED

RUTGERS UNIVERSITY PRESS

New Brunswick, Camden, and Newark, New Jersey, and London

Library of Congress Cataloging-in-Publication Data

Names: Reed, Joel Christian, author.
Title: Landscapes of activism : civil society and HIV and AIDS care in northern
Mozambique / Joel Christian Reed.
Description: New Brunswick, New Jersey : Rutgers University Press, [2018] | Series:
Medical anthropology : health, inequality, and social justice | Includes bibliographical
references and index.
Identifiers: LCCN 2017056001 (print) | LCCN 2018010494 (ebook) | ISBN
9780813596716 (epub) | ISBN 9780813596730 (web pdf) | ISBN 9780813596709
(cloth : alk. paper) | ISBN 9780813596693 (pbk. : alk. paper)
Subjects: LCSH: AIDS (Disease)—Social aspects.
Classification: LCC RA644.A25 (ebook) | LCC RA644.A25 R436 2018 (print) |
DDC 362.19697/92009679—dc23
LC record available at https://lccn.loc.gov/2017056001

A British Cataloging-in-Publication record for this book is available from the British
Library.

∞ The paper used in this publication meets the requirements of the American
National Standard for Information Sciences—Permanence of Paper for Printed
Library Materials, ANSI Z39.48-1992.

www.rutgersuniversitypress.org

Manufactured in the United States of America

I am enormously grateful to all who helped this book happen, from friends in the field, to mentors in the academy, to family (and new friends) who convalesced me back to health upon my return home.

To Anne, Merritt, Bill, David, Andrea, James, Cris, Taz, Rowenn, Michael, Kristin, Sean, Brandt, Heather, Judy, Leo, Carlitos, Januário, Falume, António, Chila, and Fátima, none of this was possible without you.

(I learned from conducting ethnography in Africa)
"The writer should never be ashamed of staring. There is nothing that does not require his attention."
–Flannery O'Connor

I was raised in a matrilineal tribe, and so . . .

(I learned from Mom and Nan)
"You are never too old to set another goal or to dream a new dream."
–C. S. Lewis

(I learned from my Aunt)
"Contrariwise, if it was so, it might be; and if it were so, it would be; but as it isn't, it ain't. That's logic."
–Lewis Carroll

If you're reading this, I thank you too for your time and energy.

CONTENTS

FOREWORD

LENORE MANDERSON

Medical Anthropology: Health, Inequality, and Social Justice is a new series from Rutgers University Press, designed to capture the diversity of contemporary medical anthropological research and writing. The beauty of ethnography is its capacity, through storytelling, to make sense of suffering as a social experience and to set it in context. Central to our focus in this series on health, illness, and social justice, therefore, is the way in which social structures and ideologies shape the likelihood and impact of infections, injuries, bodily ruptures and disease, chronic conditions and disability, treatment and care, social repair, and death.

The brief for this series is broad. The books are concerned with health and illness, healing practices, and access to care, but the authors illustrate too the importance of context—of geography, physical condition, service availability, and income. Health and illness are social facts; the circumstances of the maintenance and loss of health are always and everywhere shaped by structural, global, and local relations. Society, culture, economy, and political organization as much as ecology shape the variance of illness, disability, and disadvantage. But as medical anthropologists have long illustrated, the relationships of social context and health status are complex. In addressing these questions, the authors in this series showcase the theoretical sophistication, methodological rigor, and empirical richness of the field while expanding a map of illness, and social and institutional life to illustrate the effects of material conditions and social meanings in troubling and surprising ways.

The books in the series move across social circumstances, health conditions, and geography, and their intersections and interactions, to demonstrate how individuals, communities, and states manage assaults on well-being. The books reflect medical anthropology as a constantly changing field of scholarship, drawing on research diversely in residential and virtual communities, clinics, and laboratories; in emergency care and public health settings; with service providers, individual healers, and households; and with social bodies, human bodies, and biologies. While medical anthropology once concentrated on systems of healing, particular diseases, and embodied experiences, today the field has expanded to include environmental disaster and war, science, technology and faith, gender-based violence, and forced migration. Curiosity about the body and its vicissitudes remains a pivot for our work, but our concerns are with the location of bodies in social life and with how social structures, temporal imperatives, and shifting exigencies shape life courses. This dynamic field reflects an ethics of the discipline to address these pressing issues of our time.

Globalization has contributed to and adds to the complexity of influences on health outcomes; it (re)produces social and economic relations that institutionalize poverty, unequal conditions of everyday life and work, and environments in which diseases increase or subside. Globalization patterns the movement and relations of peoples, technologies and knowledge, and programs and treatments; it shapes differences in health experiences and outcomes across space; it informs and amplifies inequalities at individual and country levels. Global forces and local inequalities compound and constantly load on individuals to impact on their physical and mental health and on their households and communities. At the same time, as the subtitle of this series indicates, we are concerned with questions of social exclusion and inclusion, social justice and repair, again both globally and in local settings. The books will challenge readers to reflect not only on sickness and suffering, deficit and despair, but also on resistance and restitution—on how people respond to injustices and evade the fault lines that might seem to predetermine life outcomes. While not all the books take this direction, the aim is to widen the frame within which we conceptualize embodiment and suffering.

The successful development and introduction of antiretroviral therapy (ART) shifted HIV infection from a social and biological death of those who were infected to a chronic condition. But the scale-up of ART programs, the cost of their delivery in poor countries where infection is most prevalent, the acceptance of and continued adherence to therapy and preventive behaviors, and HIV's continued stigmatization mean that HIV remains a challenge personally and at the levels of government, community, and household.

Christian Reed, in *Landscapes of Activism: Civil Society and HIV and AIDS Care in Northern Mozambique*, turns to a setting of high HIV prevalence. In the coastal town of Pemba, AIDS activists, patient-activists, and the government joined forces, promising to address the challenges around HIV—affordable medication, personal support, patient reluctance, and negative community attitudes. Donors stepped in with the resources for workshops, income-generation projects, employment opportunities, and outreach. Specialist AIDS clinics were set up and began to roll out ART and support people subject to social exclusion as well as poor health. But slowly—perhaps inevitably—activism was weakened by the bureaucratic demands of the state and international development agencies. Auditing and accountability increasingly determined the roles of activists as their leaders began to concentrate on competition for prestige, personal opportunity, and cash resources. Consequently, activism was unmade. The clinics closed as national health policy took a new turn toward strengthening health systems and integrating chronic care. By the end of the *Landscapes of Activism*, the NGO with which Reed worked, Caridade, had collapsed, its leaders battling their own demons and distorted ambitions. We are left with the specter of notebooks, pens, and pencils—bought for educational interventions—that leaked into local markets; drunken leaders and disheartened patients; and community gardens turned into weeds and empty chicken runs. The dilemma is one of innovation and civil society, sustainability and the state—how to best respond to public interest and support human rights to best meet the needs of people directly affected by HIV while also tackling poverty, social vulnerability, and local and global inequalities.

INTRODUCTION
The Eye of Fátima

"My husband was a big drunk. We point to him as an example of how *not* to behave," Fátima replied to my question concerning people in her support group who stop taking their HIV medications. Fátima was HIV positive and the president of her group, *Ajuda à Próxima* (Help Your Neighbor), the second "AIDS association" established in Cabo Delgado Province in 2006. The group was a recipient of project donations from the government in the form of farming implements, seeds for planting, a plot of land, several goats, and a chicken coop. Fátima's husband, also HIV infected, had recently died. "He was on a drinking binge," she told me. "[He would] leave home early, and come home late. He stopped [treatment] for twenty-seven days before he finally died last January. He had the human right to *not* take his pills, you know." I frequently heard seemingly out-of-place "human rights" statements like this in Pemba. One person told me he had the human right for the government to buy him a house and give him a monthly stipend for being HIV positive. Another said he had the human right to divorce his wives, which he had done on seven separate occasions, each time marrying a younger woman and paying the appropriate bride price. This reflected a common belief that sex with a virgin could cure someone of HIV infection—and a unique view on the purpose of "rights talk."

Fátima continued, "Now that he's gone, I'm doing my own experiment." I leaned forward a little. "My health is improving and my CD4 is normal," she said, "and I don't miss a single pill. Sex with my husband was reinfecting me! It made my viral load increase, and I felt sicker. Without our sex together, I've had no reinfection and am starting to feel better." It took me a moment to realize that the experiment she referred to concerned chastity, and I didn't challenge her conclusions. "But there are always problems, you know. The problem now is that these pills make me forget things all of the time." She glanced down at her cell phone and keys resting on the glass table between us as if she was worried about them and then looked back up at me.

Patients often complained about medication side effects. Forgetfulness isn't all that common but is probably preferable to other common problems, such as persistent fatigue or nausea. Seated with Fátima in the lobby of Hotel Cabo Delgado on comfortable chairs, it seemed we were far from her village, about twenty kilometers away. My interviews with others in her support group occurred on wooden stools in their abandoned chicken coop, which was isolated enough to be a safe place to answer questions about HIV from an inquisitive white foreigner. The now-empty chicken coop, the missing goats, and the overgrown plot of land that produced no food were all evidence of failed support group projects, hardly morale boosters for patients who had hoped, as the promise went, to "generate" their own income.

I had heard a lot about Fátima. She was locally considered a great leader. Several members of her AIDS association told me she had saved their lives, taught them how important it was to take the pills, and encouraged them to have patience with their families and others in the community who "talked bad" about HIV and the people who had it. Fátima was in Pemba City (Cabo Delgado's provincial capital) for a government-hosted training to educate support group leaders on the new "Law 12/2009," which was related to the rights and responsibilities of people living with HIV and AIDS in Mozambique (República de Moçambique 2009). There had been many training courses for AIDS associations at that time in an effort to manage the burgeoning number of such groups in the country. When I first came to Pemba in 2007, there was one AIDS association in the province. Two years later, there were twelve officially registered with the government; several others were attempting to become registered.

From one perspective, the new law seemed well timed, coming along with government efforts to distribute treatment in more clinic facilities and locations than ever before. From another perspective, the law was just barely catching up. Article 4 of Law 12/2009 guaranteed the right to free treatment in the country, but antiretroviral medication (ARVs) had already become much more accessible over the past five or six years in places far from the capital city of Maputo—places like Pemba in the provinces. This was sped along through the "day hospitals" or HIV/AIDS-specific treatment facilities with their own pharmacies, health care staff, and waiting areas. Another component of Law 12/2009 required patients to comply with their treatment regimens. That stipulation may sound reasonable, but it was hardly enforceable given the complex factors associated with adherence to medication.

Just then, Fátima said something else unexpected: "You know, [HIV] patients go and fuck whoever. The association has a big problem with this—policing sex. You just can't monitor these things; it's too difficult." On the table between us, her cell phone buzzed and she excused herself to take the call. After a quick discussion, she put it down again and said, "This man who keeps calling . . . he wanted to 'cleanse' me after they buried my husband. I was freed from this tradition because of my HIV status. Everybody knows about this, but this man, he still wants to try anyway." Widow cleansing is practiced in parts of Africa (Kotanyi and Krings-Ney 2009). It involves sexual activity between one or more relatives of the dead man and the surviving wife in an effort to stake a claim and break the spiritual bond or any remaining supernatural attachment between the dead man and his wife. "Normally, anyone who wanted to pay could have done this. There were many of them. I took some men to the hospital and did a [HIV] test for them so they would stop asking, but this one [on the phone], he won't stop." I asked no further questions about this. No other interview participants had mentioned widow cleansing, but then again, Fátima was not a typical interview participant. Completely comfortable and unreserved, she was also the largest Mozambican woman I had ever met, easily weighing more than 230 pounds—a desirable feature for many men. A decade ago HIV was known as "the thinning disease" in southern Africa. Treatment has certainly changed that classification. Not only do people generally retain their weight, but they often gain some (another side effect of the pills).

Her cell phone buzzed again, and she picked it up to type a message. "Now most people use condoms to do the cleansing or just let the sperm fall outside of the female," she stated rather lackadaisically, distracted and staring at the phone screen. She locked eyes with me again. "Women are weaker than men, you know? Biologically, our CD4 is very undeveloped . . . We all suffer a lot. My husband's CD4 was always lower than mine, but I had more symptoms. I never understood this." The interview was almost over. "You should keep going with your reports. Tell them there in your country that we want a vaccine. The government has to find a cure so that our children don't grow up with this virus."

I thanked her and began to pack up my things when Fátima cast her gaze on a man who had just come up the stairs and was looking around the lobby. She said good-bye to me, got up, and went to greet him. This was the man who had been calling and texting her, the one who had wanted to "cleanse" her back in February. They started together down the stairs to leave the hotel, and I couldn't help wondering if this was some sort of date. I noticed then she had left her keys and phone on the table. Her side effects must have kicked in again. I picked up the items, shouted her name, and ran down the stairs after her. As I handed them over, she smiled at me one last time before they went out onto the street.

Fátima's husband, Marcos, had been a cofounder of Ajuda à Próxima the year prior, in 2008. They had started the support group together, facilitated meetings, and recruited new members. Trained in how to conduct home-based care for other people with HIV and a regular attendee at the day hospital, he was aware of what would happen to him when he ceased to take his pills. He and Fátima had come to the revelation about their condition together and saw rapid improvement in their health as they began their pharmaceutical treatment. Not even Fátima could explain why Marcos did what he did. It wasn't for lack of food, the most common complaint patients have—Mieze is a farming village. It wasn't poor clinic access—health care staff, aware of what he was doing, had even brought pills to his front door.

Marcos's decision didn't appear rational, but it was very intentional. He had *let* the virus kill him. Everyone, including Fátima, watched it happen, but they couldn't change his mind. With all the support available to him—the clinic, the group, and his own activist wife—what else could possibly have been done to save this man's life? Perhaps the prime suspect in his death was the *nipa* he drank constantly as his health slipped away—the clear, corn-based moonshine that is a cheap and available option in towns and villages all over Mozambique. In Caridade, the AIDS association with which I worked most closely, in Pemba City, I saw the same process unfold with numerous group leaders and members.

The nipa, however, points to a broader set of problems and social determinants of health that medicine can't adequately address—loss of hope, feelings of inadequacy, and internalized stigma and stress. The patient reflects these and embodies them, serving as a living representation, an example of society's challenges to care for itself. They are the "suffering body of the city" (Marcis and Inggs 2004: 453). It has become obvious that HIV treatment access—the main demand in the AIDS world of activism—is not sufficient for a total restoration of health for some patients. Biomedicine has its limits, and the dissemination of *some* kinds of moral messages needs to accompany it in order to move beyond them.

Morality and behavior are sensitive topics for anthropologists, who look upon the deployment of certain terms, images, and concepts with immense skepticism—particularly if they result in the molding of populations into efficient and adaptable subjects. We had to be careful about this, especially at first in the AIDS era. The imposition of risk categories—homosexual, Haitian, poor, African—threatened to displace needed attention to structural violence (Farmer 2006). There was a strong sense that people were getting blamed for being victims in the early days of the pandemic (Sabatier and Renee 1987). Anything less than treatment access—getting drugs into bodies—was viewed as woefully inadequate. Just prevention, just education, or just trainings were considered mere distractions.

Now that there is widespread consensus on the feasibility of scaling up treatment and providing universal coverage, it is clear that the support group, as its own intervention, has been left behind. Billions of dollars have been garnered for global health—almost U.S.$230 billion since the year 2000 (IHME 2015)—much of it to help save lives from HIV. Compared with the rise of multinational institutions such as UNAIDS and initiatives such as the President's Emergency Plan for AIDS Relief (PEPFAR), entailing massive flows of personnel and technical assistance, it is troubling that a basic model for an effective HIV support group remains elusive.

The Mozambican AIDS associations are an interesting case study because they could have been more effective—state and donor involvement, and even some AIDS activists, made them much less so. By the time AIDS associations were well established, in 2006 and 2007, antiretroviral therapy (ART) was increasingly available in Mozambican clinics. Patients did not join AIDS associations because it was a requirement or even because they feared death. Patients joined AIDS associations because they wanted, or had been promised, not just treatment but something *extra*—involvement in a project, a handout or payout, a job or a salary.

These associations were wondrously ambiguous. They were supposed to act a little like NGOs but also as spaces for emotional support and advice. They were supposed to apply for project funding but also be self-sustaining and collect membership dues and fees. They were supposed to create their own action plans, set goals, and adhere to fiscal budgets. Yet they also had to deliver on the demands of their partners, provide cheap labor, and answer to the needs of international NGOs or state programs, which in some cases relied upon them for data collection and service delivery. They were supposed to be open to anybody for membership but remain patient-centered and choose leaders to make decisions for them in a presumed atmosphere of egalitarianism.

The bureaucracy involved in running and participating in an AIDS association was reasonable for a secondary-school-educated Mozambican but just complicated enough to preclude subsistence farmers or those living in isolated, rural areas from getting involved and seeing any tangible results. Some members got paid; others did not. The interactions that occurred at the group level generated solidarity, along with greed and jealousy. Mozambican AIDS associations were not shining examples of either civil society or a therapeutic community, yet they contained the seeds of both. They were uniquely Mozambican, pieced together from components of a socialist past and nominally "of the people," yet they also hearkened to the global community of HIV-positive patients that social scientists praised as naturally occurring, ubiquitous, and unstoppable.

Anthropologists studying HIV have begun to note the trouble with portraying civil society as utopian (Bähre 2007; Marsland 2012; Marcis 2012). Initial enthusiasm about patients coming together in protest against poor drug availability and perceived unfair government policies sparked a high level of interest in the concept of social solidarity. Famous examples of this emerged in the headlines and drew worldwide attention—the AIDS Coalition to Unleash Power (ACT UP) in the United States and the Treatment Action Campaign (TAC) in South Africa—that portrayed people with HIV as a united front, politically combative ideologues formed and shaped by overly bureaucratic institutions whose inaction was letting people die unnecessarily.

To describe the phenomenon, theorists latched onto the idea of *biosociality*, a concept that emphasizes patient mobilization and highlights the formation and activity of groups of people who identify with one another based on a common genetic or biomedical illness. Patients latched onto the idea of human rights, positioning treatment as foundational to the physical and mental well-being of high numbers of people and thus covered under international treaties and agreements, of which most African nations are signatories. The struggle for HIV treatment, in this light, was a political one, a function of overcoming stigma and seeking inclusivity in health care and government programs.

The HIV support group was supposed to be a breeding ground for this approach. It was intended as a site for the stimulation of demand for care and the realization of benefits owed to affected persons on the part of states and institutions responsible for their protection and welfare. From this perspective, it is social recognition, from the state or similar authority, which mitigates powerlessness. It is social recognition that legitimates the person and his or her group, drawing attention to the issue and inviting concern, assistance, and intervention. Social science has labeled this *biological citizenship* (Rose and Novas 2005; Petryna 2013), the claiming of resources as recompense for a chronic illness through appealing to objective or expert evaluation in order to save lives or meet basic needs.

The results of this can manifest in a number of different ways. In a perfect world, it would level the playing field, allowing those most severely impacted to live as healthily as possible. It would point to the fruits of patient advocacy, overturning misconceptions and dispelling ignorance. It would also legitimate efforts at empowerment and facilitate fellowship among those affected. HIV-positive support groups were supposed to be the site for the practical application of activism, holding government accountable, taking charge of their lives, managing the impressions that others have about them, and offsetting stigma. In the popular imagination, these groups came to be recognized as something both old and new, civil society but with humanitarian features, a privileged kind of social movement, deserving of encouragement and even financial support—if they fulfilled the roles set out for them.

This book is primarily about the dysfunction of AIDS associations, the utility of rights-based demands, and calls for social transformation. Expectations about political AIDS activism first made patienthood cogent and then led to yet another example of "dysappearing bodies" (Imrie 2005: 98)—patients appear to disappear into the framework of national health systems, becoming voiceless. Once taken for granted and now highly visible everywhere, AIDS activists have now demanded themselves out of existence, barely able to claim special privileges anymore. AIDS activism, its short-term goals and its consumability and expendable nature, manifested itself in Mozambique as just another kind of "governmentality" (Lemke 2001; Ingram 2010; Foucault 2010), allowing for the imposition of certain morals, attitudes, and modes of living onto entire groups of people without their obvious and active consent. Gone, consequently, are the grassroots "movements." Still remaining are the multinational institutions and bureaucracies that rose up around them.

Now part of an antiquated system, the Mozambican AIDS associations never really achieved what they wanted, which was to participate in the HIV/AIDS "industry" and to be fully vested in the programs taking place around, for, and with them. They were provided a model with which to do this, and it did not suffice. The reasons are informed by the contours of history and the parameters of a global health industry that leaves no corner of the world untouched. During my time with Caridade[1]—the group that took me in, allowing me to live and work with them as if I were a member myself—AIDS activism in Mozambique rose and fell, decidedly, in relation to the demands of the state. This challenges the idea that involvement in activism is liberating or counterhegemonic. While these beliefs are deep-seated and rooted in history, by better understanding Caridade and groups like it, a broader understanding of what activism "does" for people is possible, even in a low-income (or "less-developed") state like Mozambique.

A DEVELOPING NATION?

Mozambique ranks 181 out of 187 on the United Nations Human Development Index (UNDP 2016), a low position shared with South Sudan. A country of twenty-eight million people, life expectancy is about fifty-five years. Little more than half of Mozambicans (59 percent) are literate, and there is a 69 percent primary-school dropout rate.[2] The population in multidimensional poverty[3] is 70 percent and 90 percent of working Mozambicans make less than $3.10 per day. According to the IMF (2014), agriculture provides a living for almost 80 percent of Mozambicans; efforts to reduce poverty were strong in the immediate postwar period (after 1992) but have since tapered off. Mozambique faces serious challenges regarding gender equality. Though parliament is composed of 40 percent women, maternal mortality is high and so is teenage pregnancy, ranking Mozambique 139 out of 159 countries on the Gender Inequality Index. Mozambique also has one of the worst global shortages of human resources for health, with only three doctors and twenty-one nurses per one hundred thousand inhabitants.

During the 1990s, after the end of protracted colonial and civil wars, Mozambique became a darling of the international development (and business) communities. An influx of NGOs, loans from the World Bank and IMF, and private sector investment saw the economy rise on average of 4.73 percent per capita per year. Recently, this has waned. The country is now facing the possibility of a debilitating debt crisis related to secretive bank loans the government took out amounting to more than one billion dollars (Quinn 2016). Once hailed as a shining example of "Africa rising," a counternarrative of development failure in Mozambique is quickly becoming well established (Brooks 2017).

A lack of optimism around HIV/AIDS may similarly be unfolding. Mozambique has the fifth largest HIV epidemic in sub-Saharan Africa, and prevalence recently rose from 11.5 percent in 2009 to 13.2 percent in 2015 (INS 2015). The difference is more pronounced in select provinces, including Cabo Delgado, where most of the research for this book occurred. From 2009 to 2015, prevalence in Cabo Delgado increased from 9.5 percent (one of the lowest in the country) to 13.8 percent (hovering around the national average). An estimated 1.5 million people in Mozambique are living with HIV, and modeled data suggests that 223 new infections and 108 deaths occur per day (UNAIDS 2016b). There is some good news—the number of HIV-positive persons on antiretroviral therapy (ART) has increased over the years. Almost a million adults (990,000) were estimated to be enrolled in treatment programs in the country in 2016, or roughly 65 percent, versus just 13 percent in 2009 (MISAU 2017a).

But these numbers eclipse some important undercurrents, including tension between humanitarian NGOs and better-financed global initiatives like PEPFAR. In chapter 5, I will problematize these apparent treatment gains in several ways. Significant declines around HIV knowledge and awareness indicate the disease's momentum is not decelerating. Continuing foreign aid and "intervention" is still needed, raising questions about national sovereignty and lingering dependence.

Undoubtedly, one of Mozambique's most serious problems is how members of the ruling party benefit disproportionally from development aid when compared to the general population (Cunguara and Hanlon 2012). Though Mozambique is nominally democratic and held up as an international success story, big projects backed by foreign investors play questionable key roles in relationships and national improvement schemes. The openness to global capitalism that the country displays is anchored in industry (Gisselquist, Pérez Niño, and Le Billon 2014) and partnership with China (Alden and Chichava 2014) in ways that are environmentally harmful and do not lift the masses out of poverty. Power is concentrated in the hands of an elite few, allowing Mozambique to create hundreds of millionaires at a rate that rivals that of any other African country. All this has occurred despite the nation's failure to meet any of the Millennium Development Goals (Brooks 2017). In chapter 2, I will discuss in depth Mozambique's history—the wars and now privatization—and how this dovetails with the potential of a free and fair civil society in the form of the AIDS associations and the HIV-positive persons who formerly comprised them.

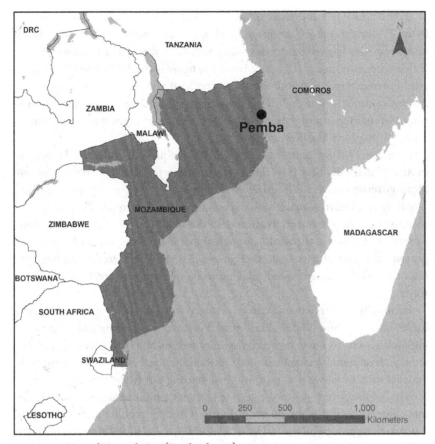

FIGURE I.1. Map of Mozambique (Pemba shown)

CHAPTER OUTLINE

In chapter 1, "Studying HIV and HIV-Positive People," I provide an overview of HIV/AIDS from an anthropological perspective and discuss the methods used to collect my data and write this ethnography. Despite humanity's best efforts, the virus remains a sustained pandemic and a threat that transcends conventional biomedical thought, imposing itself on our social worlds and marking the recent era of globalization. Since its "discovery" in the 1980s, HIV has taken many lives as well as the time and resources of researchers and charities attempting to prevent and treat it. An important aspect of the global response to HIV involved civil society reactions. People with AIDS (PWAs), as a social category, emerged from identity politics, with the earliest examples of activism entrenched in gay rights and demands for medical equality and quicker progress.

By the time AIDS activism exploded in southern Africa, coalescing famously in the Treatment Action Campaign (TAC), social scientists had already helped implode misleading risk categories—like homosexual or Haitian—and HIV was widely recognized as a social justice issue. The figure of the AIDS activist was powerful and inspiring, paving the way for greater treatment access, especially on the African continent. Though AIDS activism is now in decline—an effect of its perceived strength and momentum—the need for resilient support groups remains, especially in places like Mozambique.

Chapter 2, "'Movements' of the Past: Mozambique, Caridade, and Treatment in Africa," discusses how HIV came to be an important concern to the Mozambican government and how AIDS associations became part of the response. Not long ago, international health experts urged caution in administering HIV treatment on the continent. Treatment in the public sector was withheld from patients in this part of the world, out of fear that locals would be unable to comply with complex pharmaceutical regimens. As AIDS activists carried out protests and NGOs implemented pilot projects, hesitation to treat Africans was waylaid.

Eventually, HIV treatment access was placed squarely on the agendas of global health initiatives and NGOs alike. Interest grew for supporting and even creating such groups to serve as the community face of HIV and encourage others to begin treatment. In chapter 2, I introduce Caridade, a support group for HIV patients that, when we first met, was just starting out in Pemba City. Medical NGOs and the government were keen to partner with Caridade, providing funding, office space, and other resources. Ideally, Caridade would flourish like other AIDS activist groups before it. But in Mozambique, relations between the state and civil society are fraught with tension. A history of centralized power in this postcommunist country makes voluntary associations between and among citizens difficult to take hold and evolve.

Chapter 3, "AIDS Associations in Cabo Delgado Province," highlights the institutional and organizational features of Mozambican AIDS activism. Pemba City's first HIV/AIDS support group, Caridade, is located in the heart of its busiest neighborhood. The office functions as a kind of drop-in center for people seeking help with an HIV diagnosis, and the group grew quickly in influence and reputation. Initially funded by a single NGO, other partners began to take notice and employ Caridade leaders and members in their community health projects. There was some pressure on the group to conform to outside expectations in terms of collecting and reporting data, adhering to financial policies and requirements, and adapting or modifying the group's goals and objectives.

Delving into everyday life with the group revealed new partnerships and funding to be a grand source of division and conflict. Meetings could be difficult, especially when the group no longer seemed to provide support to one another or those who rely on it for help. Amid nostalgic talk of Caridade's glory days, new HIV support groups began to form and splinter off, especially to take advantage of new donor money available for AIDS civil society. The state response to this growing civil society amounted to an attempt at control and standardization. Policies and procedures were instituted for such groups to register for formal status. In the swirl of trainings and workshops designed to capacitate civil society, the activities of groups were diverted and redirected. Paradoxically, this unfortunate outcome served as justification for greater state and NGO involvement, as civil society appeared to need help because it functioned less well than expected.

Chapter 4, "Challenges to HIV/AIDS Activism in the 'Subuniverse' of Cabo Delgado," highlights the community-oriented features of AIDS activism. Most publicity on and about AIDS activists is generated from urban or cosmopolitan settings. But in northern Mozambique, the most common type of activist was not particularly well educated or politically oriented. Patient-activists in isolated areas seek different kinds of resources and benefits; their aesthetic tastes and practical needs are not the same as those in larger towns and cities. Patient-activists described here occupied a unique existence, a "subuniverse" of the activist dimension. They related to one another and to those around them in ways that did not contribute to the preferred narrative embraced and espoused by mainstream, urban, globally aware AIDS activists.

As a result, the challenges faced here went undisclosed and were poorly acknowledged. HIV patients continued to face problems that in other settings may have been dealt with more comprehensively. Due to stigma, some were afraid to live openly and did not discuss the virus with others. Due to poor education, myths and opinions about HIV and its transmission circulated unimpeded and remained poorly addressed. Programs staffed and run by people with HIV did not function independently and relied heavily on state and NGO technical assistance. Alcoholism was rampant yet not discussed, and many patients dropped out or could not comply, with treatment programs. Despite lengthy and sustained attention to the medical needs of HIV patient and activists, a sound model for addressing basic emotional and psychological concerns remained elusive.

Chapter 5, "the (Dis)integration of the Day Hospitals," highlights the political dimensions of HIV activism in Mozambique. The nationwide closure of "day hospitals," or AIDS clinics, resulted in downgraded services, drug stockouts, and diminished treatment access. Activists responded with organized street protests and by picketing government offices. Their anger was directed toward the country's minister of health, who claimed the facilities were wasteful, unnecessary, and unsustainable. While the protests pitted patients against their own government, the day hospital closures did not happen in a vacuum. Similar changes were occurring in other developing countries geared toward integrating disease-specific services into national health systems. Evaluated against this backdrop, the traditional tactic of AIDS activists—to enact localized protests—had no effect. Their primary demands, to provide treatment for all, were already adopted by the wider international community, undermining the activist cause and dispersing the power and clarity of the patient voice.

The AIDS activists' mistake was focusing too heavily on medicine and pills as opposed to tightly knit communities and associations. Chapter 5 exposes the tension and debate around "health systems strengthening," identifying as the winners not civil society but political and governmental elites. Close examination of the AIDS activist community in Mozambique, after health systems strengthening, reveals a loss of momentum, intense competition and careerism, and an accompanying deflation of purpose and vision. Having already degenerated to the level of "slacktivism" through half-hearted advocacy and minimal support for ordinary HIV patients, the efficacy and authenticity of AIDS activism in Mozambique appears to have come to an end.

The final chapter, "Biosocial Governmentality," points out that activism's effects on ordinary support groups were much less empowering than imagined. The theoretical concept of biosociality—a shared social consciousness based on a disease diagnosis—has brought attention to patient groups, but political involvement made them a target for the market and paved the way for dissolution. I discuss how Caridade fizzled out and unraveled, becoming a source of prestige and income for just a few of its more prominent members. HIV patient groups in Africa qualified as a site for experimentation in the world of global health. What should have been a thriving point of contact bridging the lay-expert divide instead became a source of cheap NGO labor and the logical place for gauging potential receptivity to expand pharmaceutical markets in developing nations.

Activism, by trafficking in the same language and currency as the institutions it claims to challenge—demands, recognition, and power—is just as capable of shaping mood and desire as any other art of governance, stripping patient groups of their diversity and compromising alternative models. Considering a greater variety of sources as examples of biosociality, researchers can help fix this problem. High-level donors and funders still call for greater patient involvement. There is still a need for patient groups to improve adherence and inspire hope for people at risk of being lost to the system. AIDS activism, perhaps in a different, more practical and accessible form, may have an additional role to play in the future.

ABBREVIATIONS, FOREIGN WORDS, AND OTHER TERMS

ACT UP   AIDS Coalition to Unleash Power

AIDS   Acquired Immune Deficiency Syndrome

ANC   African National Congress

ART   Antiretroviral Therapy

ARVs   Antiretrovirals, Antiretroviral pills or medication

Associativismo   Portuguese for the concept of civil society associations (lit. associationism)

Bairro   Portuguese for neighborhood, an area of a city or town

Barraca   A small roadside or neighborhood store, selling dry goods, alcohol, batteries, and other items

Caridade   Fictitious name of the main HIV/AIDS support group in the book; means "charity" in Portuguese.

Capulana   Local cloth, spectacularly patterned and typically used by women for waist and head wraps

CD4+   T-cells, helper cells, and also refers to a common laboratory test (CD4 count)

CDC   Centers for Disease Control and Prevention

CNCS   *Conselho Nacional de Combate ao SIDA* (Mozambique's National AIDS Council)

day hospital   *Hospital de dia*, AIDS clinics tailored specifically to that patient population

Desafio Jovem   Youth Challenge (in Portuguese), an AIDS association and local health NGO

Doencas incognitas   unknown diseases in Portuguese

DREAM   Mozambique's first AIDS treatment program, run by Catholic charities and the Community of Saint Egidio

EGPAF   Elizabeth Glazer Pediatric AIDS Foundation

Frelimo   Frente de Libertação de Moçambique (Mozambique Liberation Front, Mozambique's ruling party)

GHIs   Global Health Initiatives (such as PEPFAR or Global Fund)

HDD   Day hospital, *hospital de dia* in Portuguese

HSS   Health Systems Strengthening, a collection of policies purportedly channeling funds for HIV/AIDS into government budgets and multinational programs

HIV Human Immunodeficiency Virus

Kidudu Makua word for HIV. "Kidudu grande" (big HIV) also used as the virus progresses.

Liga Contra Discriminação Antidiscrimination League in Portuguese

MATRAM Mozambican Access to Treatment Movement

MISAU *Ministério de Saúde* (Mozambican Ministry of Health)

MONASO Mozambican Network of AIDS Service Organizations, a government NGO

MSF Médecins Sans Frontières, or Doctors Without Borders

Nipa cheap, strong, corn-based, home-brewed moonshine

NGO Nongovernmental organization

Núcleos *Núcleos Provinciais de Combate à Sida* (Provincial AIDS Offices)

PALS Positive and Living Squad

PEN *Plano Estratégico Nacional de Combate ao HIV/SIDA* (Mozambique's National Strategic Plan to Combat HIV/AIDS)

PEPFAR President's Emergency Plan for AIDS Relief (an American AIDS treatment initiative)

PHC Primary health care

PWAs People with AIDS

RENSIDA *Rede Nacional das Pessoas Vivendo com HIV/SIDA* (National Association of People Living with HIV/AIDS)

UNAIDS Joint United Nations Programme on HIV/AIDS

USAID United States Agency for International Development

TAC Treatment Action Campaign

TRIPS The Agreement on Trade-Related Aspects of Intellectual Property Rights

Vergonha Stigma, or shame

WHO World Health Organization

LANDSCAPES OF ACTIVISM

1 · STUDYING HIV AND HIV-POSITIVE PERSONS

HIV, as we have come to know it, is much more than a just a virus or infectious disease. Despite global efforts, it remains a sustained pandemic, and HIV is a term loaded with social and cultural meaning. Ever since HIV was "discovered" in the early 1980s, it has been at the center of medical and moral controversy. It has altered the world, forcing us to rethink science in everyday life, spurring divisions and revelations about what disease "is." HIV has clarified some very important realities—namely, that we live our lives interconnected, among webs of circumstance, and within multiple networks of institutions, persons, and political negotiations that affect life directly, whether we like it or not.

This recognition of complex interdependency occurred first in scientific and activist circles and eventually in international concerns for global health. One main lesson—that HIV won't just go away—is written in blood, with an estimated seventy million infections and thirty-five million AIDS deaths since the epidemic began (UNAIDS 2016). The virus presents as a biomarker for globalization and demonstrates how health is mutually and collectively shaped. HIV reminds us that living and dying are graphed alongside myriad other social relations, ones that overlap and coconstitute both tragedy and hope, depending on circumstances and who is willing to help. How much support people have, how much money, and how much access to information about their illness become important concerns to offset the effects of the virus. Conventional biomedical thought—that HIV is simply a virus and nothing more—seems either naïve or a reductionist assertion, imposing sanctions upon the more open social terrains capable of operating against this tenacious threat.

HIV, especially at first, highlighted a lack of sovereignty over our own bodies. There was no treatment, so the virus appeared unstoppable. Those who became infected were unable to dispute the inevitable disruption to their lives, unable to take back the territory they once had—their own cells and DNA—against an enemy barely known or visible. Even now with treatment, the virus, as one of the fastest known evolving entities, combats the drugs we design. So along with those personally affected, the global health community remains locked in a war with HIV. Because of what gets lost, the war metaphor, though overplayed, is an apt one. Apart from robbing our physical bodies and disrupting our dreams and futures, the virus has consumed the time and intellectual talents of many researchers, bureaucrats, philanthropists, charities, and politicians. We like to think now that the conflict is stable, yet on how people can best survive the virus and help others do so too, better data and guidance remain constant concerns.

Continual "war" and the need for more data are two dependable continuities, but there is at least one other: epidemiological and international development work continue to construct the "facts" of this disease so that the virus and its parameters remain politically and socially determined. HIV was not always called HIV, it changed names several times.[1] Surveillance definitions were too narrow, then got expanded.[2] Calculations and models estimating global and local burdens were modified in response to changing methods of data collection.[3] CD4 counts and other thresholds for treatment were altered and grew more inclusive (Bor et al. 2017). These shifts were presented as part of a routine process, as trying to keep pace with science. But many were influenced by activist concerns, responses to mistakes, and legal actions.

The latest change that has occurred relates to defunding HIV-specific interventions, diverting funds toward states and their health systems. This too is presented as imperative, as a response to good data, yet consensus has emanated from the same sources as always—experts and governmental elites who, at least in Mozambique, have yet to keep many promises. Since "health systems strengthening" (HSS) began in Mozambique, HIV rates have risen, while prevention and knowledge about the virus have not (INS 2015). The lack of sovereignty now, the new war on AIDS, is a struggle over memory, past and future, which, like science and medicine, is open to negotiation. Like the virus itself, the history of HIV evolves quickly. It must be remembered; otherwise, we will not continue to get as far, as quickly. Other common infectious diseases have never captured the attention that HIV has—though maybe another will one day. For now, despite many claims to the contrary, HIV remains exceptional.

Anthropologists and social scientists have contributed to the HIV/AIDS narrative in a variety of ways. Approaches included mapping its social dimensions and the ways it moves within and through particular societies (Farmer 2006; Fassin 2007), performing research related to prevention or medical intervention (Green and Ruark 2011), and compiling testimonies and theories in the midst of crisis (Bastos 2002). Anthropologists have studied the response to AIDS in specific categories such as homosexuals (Brummelhuis 2004), drug users (Singer 2005), and women (Chase 2011). Social scientists have contextualized the epidemic in geographical contexts requiring a good deal of cultural introspection—for example, in Africa (Crane 2013), Brazil (Biehl and Eskerod 2009), and India (Hollen 2013). Anthropologists have engaged activist communities (Iliffe 2006) and the medical and public health professions (Pfeiffer and Chapman 2010). Researchers have explored sexuality and relationships in regard to the virus (Hirsch et al. 2010), debated its place in global capitalism (Petryna, Lakoff, and Kleinman 2006), and contributed to ethical discussions concerning methodology, theory, and practice (Parker and Ehrhardt 2001). These additions to HIV/AIDS knowledge were perhaps unexpected by the medical research community when social scientists initially became involved. Notably, anthropologists did not analyze only risk behavior. Instead, we told and continue to tell stories that otherwise would have never been brought to light.

An important aspect of the global response to HIV involves civil society reactions, which have impacts on various other fronts (Rau 2006). Influencing scientific investigation, the evolution of therapy, and the conception and implementation of policies at all levels was a loose "social movement." Given its origins, it exceeded expectations and became an interesting feature of how the pandemic played out in almost every context. AIDS activism begs examination as a social movement primarily to understand how society handles an enormous medical problem. There are other examples of social *reactions* to large epidemics—such as leprosy (Plagerson 2005), yellow fever (Nuwer 2009), and cholera (Ross 2015)—but nothing on a scale similar to HIV.

What was different about AIDS activism was its origin among patient bases, which previously formed only sporadically and for much less stigmatized diseases. As AIDS activists drew on reference points already in use by similar support and self-help groups, such as those championing black power and feminism (Livingston, McAdoo, and Mills 2010), the nature of AIDS activism grew and became further politicized. Other blueprints, which helped AIDS activism evolve in this way, included resistance to racism and apartheid (Powers 2012).

People with AIDS (PWAs), as a social category subject to academic study, has roots in early AIDS activism and can be traced back to its initial articulation in New York City during the late '80s and early '90s (Chambré 2006; France 2016). The term was initially associated with identity politics and linked to the creation of the first groups of people that organized themselves around a seropositive status. The Gay Men's Health Crisis (GMHC), the People with AIDS Coalition, and ACT UP helped facilitate community research initiatives through the lens of PWAs as a group open to targeted intervention. Awareness campaigns and community support initiatives gave rise to collaboration with government entities, scientific institutes, and pharmaceutical companies (Epstein 1996).

On the other coast of the United States, in California, parallel and similar institutions evolved in Los Angeles and San Francisco (Roth 2017). Project Inform came into being as an alternative to slow and ineffective medical investigations, especially the slow approval of drugs by the FDA, and led to splinter groups like the AIDS Foundation and the Healing Alternatives Foundation. Other urban centers benefitted from this proliferation of activism, most notably Boston, Washington, Philadelphia, Chicago, and Toronto, where sizable communities of ACT UP and similar associations of people with AIDS began demanding better services and medical attention. A few years later every state in the United States had some presence of AIDS activists and organizations. Countries in Europe, and Australia, developed their own versions (Carter and Watney 1997). These included the Terrence Higgins Trust and the Body Positive in London, AIDES in Paris, and Deutsche AIDS Hilfe in Berlin. On an organizational level, these groups expanded beyond linking sufferers with health services. Technical assistance for other groups and organizations just starting out became a focused mission, including the transfer of experiences through civil rights (rather than just gay rights), the language of democracy, and economic prosperity.

These models carried over in developing nations, the clearest example being South Africa's TAC. However, in new democracies, where civil and postcolonial difficulties had lasting effects, the consolidation of activism was impacted. In less-developed countries, poverty limited the capacity for the organic growth of independent and outspoken groups. Languages of individual rights and citizenship took center stage, and activism grew in an environment of collaboration with development agencies and other external forces geared toward fighting the pandemic. A common human rights language was adopted under the influence of international institutions. African AIDS activism gained momentum mostly through claims for the human right to health care, positioning patients as vulnerable to world capitalist economics and states as failing or uncaring. This coalesced succinctly in TAC, where social activism combined with global humanitarianism with the common goal of providing medication to those with no access to it (Grebe 2011).

What TAC and African support groups inherited from prior activist tendencies included a preference for assistance programs, concepts of buddy systems, and personal, psychological, or practical guidance (Robins 2006). But in most cases, people's needs could not be met only at the local level. Success was more quickly found in collaborating with umbrella groups, leading to the formation of national networks. In this way, old priorities were redefined and new ones created. The vocation of groups and the assistance they desired began to include home-based care (Kalofonos 2014), especially where general health services were deficient. Some groups became politicized, while others became subsumed as an NGO workforce or as labor for hospitals and the programs of multinational institutions.

In many cases, links with communities and accountability to the needs of patients ceased to be the main focus. Best practices were dominated by preexisting or imported programs of prevention. Safe sex forums, recommended modes of healthy living, and the testimonies of those living with the virus became a precondition for participation in activist circles and volunteer-type positions, where the possibility of obtaining small salaries garnered interest. Meetings and trainings became a forum for producing "patient-activists." The possibilities of basic support groups, designed mainly for lay patients, got subsumed and became undervalued.

The African HIV-positive support group, therefore, inherited and was predated by imported conceptions of who an HIV-positive person was and what he or she should be doing. The word that underscored everything was *resistance*—to not having health care or access to medication or to being outcast from a meaningful social existence. Like early AIDS activists in America and Europe, who renounced the role of victim and a passive sense of being defeated, African support groups designed around political empowerment models gained momentum. These were held up as examples, much more so than less-visible groups, and subsequently supported by funders and outside organizations (Robins 2004). Such models renounced the simple role of "patient," and required that people with the virus become specialists in their disease area. This involved contributing to scientific and medical practice and conversing in the language of international human rights.

Hence AIDS activism in African settings was a continuation of Western movements, including those focused on gay rights, women's rights, and self-esteem (Hunter 2010; Beyrer et al. 2011). The language of personal politics was similar, as was the need for freedom from oppression. The expectation was that HIV-positive persons, rather than waiting to die from AIDS, would become their own advocates. Some authors claimed that HIV-positive persons were standing up for their rights as citizens (Jones 2016), while others showed that they had nothing else to lose (Chan 2015). In some circumstances—when communities, families, and friends are sources of rejection—embracing a new or alternative social identity is welcome as a means for health care and income. This option, however, was not available to all patients, particularly those less educated or those dwelling farther from urban centers. There were groups, and some members of particular groups, for whom the practical aspects of daily survival, income or livelihood, and generally coping with being seropositive remained of prime importance. The need for and importance of the support group—as an intervention and entity all its own—was never completely lost but unfortunately remained stunted and poorly developed.

SUPPORT GROUPS AND SOCIAL JUSTICE

Illness support groups serve as an indicator species. In places where they are unavailable or in decline, our environment (our "ecosystem") is more damaged, the illness experience more estranged, and life undervalued. Where support groups proliferate, on the other hand, society tends to be freer and more democratic, mutual trust and confidence in public institutions is higher (Evans, Henry, and Sundstrom 2016). Support groups are a proxy measure for community affluence and empowerment. While ideally available to persons in crisis, to go searching for one is a very different experience in wealthier countries than in poorer countries (Kingod et al. 2017). A nation's infrastructure makes a difference; so too does attention paid to an epidemic. As a crisis crescendos, snagging headlines and raising public outcry, support groups are expected to form, especially for a chronic illness or widespread malaise. It's almost counterintuitive if they do not. Access to peer-to-peer counseling seems humane and natural and potentially very effective.

Take, for instance, the current scale of opioid and heroin abuse in the state of West Virginia (Caldwell 2017), where 86 percent of deaths in 2016 were attributed to drug overdose. Support groups are a big part of that response, especially in the face of floundering federal assistance. When science and/or politics fail to make a difference, resilient communities still do. Fostering the expansion of support groups and their maintenance, just as much as providing treatments or medical technology, therefore, entails a degree of ethical fairness. Support groups—their very existence and capacity to thrive—facilitate a process of decolonization and social justice. Insulated from politics and safe from shifting, sometimes divisive science,[4] they may be better off.

A support group is composed of people with common experiences and concerns who provide moral and emotional support for one another. They fulfill several functions—educating each other, sharing their experiences, serving as mutual sources of strength. Support groups typically form around aspects of health that are difficult to address in clinics, augmenting conventional services and in some cases serving as an adequate substitution. A powerful example is Alcoholics Anonymous, a program that has proven more effective than medical approaches for curbing addiction and preventing relapse (Scott et al. 2017).

The "anonymous" model has taken on a life of its own. It has been reproduced for other rehabilitative purposes, including gambling, hoarding, overeating, and sex addiction. Different kinds of support groups exist to address not vices but psychosocial concerns. They are commonly created for problems like bereavement, depression, suicide prevention, posttraumatic stress, and divorce. Still others are formed for people with chronic illness, such as diabetes, dementia, and HIV/AIDS (as discussed here in depth). A central concern of *Landscapes of Activism* is why HIV-positive persons who benefit from peer counseling and emotional support don't have access to strong support groups, especially in Mozambique and southern Africa.

Studies among support groups show that members are more knowledgeable than nonmembers about the causes and treatments of disorders, cope more easily with the difficulties they encounter, feel stronger, have less negative emotions, receive more social support, and are less anxious about their future (Bademli and Duman 2014). In social network theory, support groups foster access to resources, social influence, creativity and innovation, relational development, and collective action (Chewning and Montemurro 2016). The medical world consistently endorses support groups as an important source of emotional and practical support for patients (Hu 2017; Delisle et al. 2017). But despite clear benefits, the factors leading to their successful establishment and maintenance are not well understood. While community embeddedness, duration of existence, and frequency of interaction are all important variables to consider, there are few details on how people in these types of communities manage everyday life (Naoi 2017). In *Landscapes of Activism*, I attempt to contribute to this small body of knowledge through a highly contextualized study based in Pemba, Mozambique.

Working in developing nations, many anthropologists, including myself, have encountered only weak support groups operating in a constant mode of damage control. What draws patients into networks or groups in these cases is a subsistence crisis. The term "moral economy" has been used to describe support groups and other community interventions in Africa (Prince 2012), especially to illustrate how groups become infiltrated or influenced by outside forces. In this formulation, regimes of self-care are an imposition. Encouraging members to eat a balanced diet draws greater attention to hunger and poverty (Kalofonos 2010). Identities and ways of living conform to donor expectations, making groups more manageable, and fostering competition over scarce resources. Information given about HIV is sometimes perceived as manipulative, attempting to regulate sexuality, encourage condom use or abstinence, and inspiring people to "live positively" through disclosing their status to others (Benton 2015).

The ethnographic research I will discuss here does not challenge these assertions, but it does take them a step further. True, patient groups seem unable to escape biopolitical forces that draw them into NGO economies, converting them into just another programmatic intervention. But in addition, the effects of these same powerful forces convey through the concepts of political activism and advocacy, so that this too becomes a technique of neoliberal governance rather than of freedom and liberation. The support group, intended to ameliorate stigma, poverty, and feelings of powerlessness for the chronically ill, ceases to be as helpful when conflated with, or replaced by, civil society. As a result, basic medical progress, collective resistance to oppression, and social or community uplift are all the more negated, cut off, and shut down. The way through this entanglement is the establishment of support group models free from government involvement and geared soundly toward the goals of rehabilitation and posttraumatic growth. This requires broadening the normative definition of "activist-ness"—of who an activist is and what their purpose is—to include those who are not just politically engaged or globally connected but working more closely with one another in less prestigious, relatively isolated situations.

THE STRANGE DECLINE OF AIDS ACTIVISM

What is the role of HIV/AIDS activism and advocacy in the lives of patients in northern Mozambique? This book seeks to answer that question. The answer, of course, is not straightforward but lies in nuance. Much of what we know about this kind of activism is drawn from just a few sources and from the cosmopolitan, urban areas of just a few nations. Details and events like the ones I will describe here have not garnered as much interest in anthropology or development studies. On the contrary, they may even have been overlooked or dismissed. Some stories about HIV patient groups have been made available for public consumption and others have not. Because of that, the way we perceive the topic depends greatly on how it has (usually selectively) been presented.

Through news headlines, high-impact journal articles, sound bites, websites, and promotional materials, AIDS activists around the turn of the century were depicted as heroes and became an imposing force. Patient mobilization for treatment access was soon considered a transnational phenomenon. Part of that inspiration was the stereotypical figure of the AIDS activist. Demanding, deservedly antagonistic, compliant with medical regimes but noncompliant with the states and corporations who chose how and when to provide them, he or she became a juggernaut of a trope, one of almost mythical proportions.

Long-term justice, however, would require much more than just strong pride and protest marches. To become permanent fixtures as civil society intermediaries, patient groups needed greater resourcefulness and to know more about working together as a community. That struggle, a very different one, turned out to be more difficult. Groups that were apolitical or unsuccessfully able to negotiate the treacherous path toward funding and notoriety got left behind. Alternate conceptions of "activists," less educated or cosmopolitan or of a much lower profile, remained understudied. Several consequences emerged because of this. One was that medication, and not people, continued to receive the most attention. Another was the expectation that all HIV-positive people should become politically active, progressing along an imaginary ladder of cultural evolution (a classic social science fallacy).

Other consequences arose more directly from the tension between "the establishment" and perceived "troublemakers." AIDS activists had been labeled rebellious since first dropping out of clinical trials and smuggling drugs across international borders.[5] Such symbolic action, much more than the number of lives saved, contributed so successfully to the theater of revolution so as to appear as a distinct threat to global governance and economic order. As polarizing figures, in one way or another, they would have to be dealt with. From the perspective of government, industry, charities, and multilateral institutions, activists and their patient groups could continue to be divisive and problematic or be put to work.

Common ground for this was quickly found in the businesses of patient recruitment, disease surveillance, and expanding pharmaceutical markets. Serving hybrid logics, it was proposed that groups could work both for the community (as safe places for needy persons) and for the state or its proxies (looping patients into care and therapy). These combined efforts appeased international funders, local authorities, and most activists alike. But in doing this, support groups became the place not to enact a curriculum of independence and resilience but to eventually reinforce a hidden bias against activism's root inspirations. Several other options, besides confrontation, could be explored there.

And why not? The search for social and economic influence is of immense interest to everyone, including the poor and HIV positive. Besides making demands on the system, there were many other practices to consider and try to master, like grant writing, managing a nonprofit, or specializing in service delivery. That support groups would be shackled with NGOs in this endeavor was not accidental but required. Apart from NGOs (and perhaps religion or local tradition), there is no other framework for citizen participation in much of southern Africa, especially in the hinterlands of a post-Marxist, war-ravaged, resource-rich, and rapidly privatizing country like Mozambique.

Circa 2004, following MSF and TAC's efforts in the Western Cape, collaboration among patients, NGOs, and the state was suddenly the new norm. Yet nothing really changed overnight. Unsurprisingly, in anticipation of this new arrangement, the process got rushed. Some bureaucrats and even field-level workers, expecting better, were shocked to find that most patient groups had to be coaxed into existence, beguiled or encouraged with stipends, food handouts, or other incentives. Good for the short term but hardly for the long, the full potential of the support group as a force for stability was thus thwarted at the outset. As the number of groups multiplied but funding didn't, the situation inched toward patronage, meritocracy, and nepotism. The unschooled, unconnected, and powerless (the truly destitute) got pushed out soon enough. Embracing partnerships and project funding invoked important changes in the composition of support groups and altered available visions for the future.

History shows that the activist critique gets blunted according to how likely they are to garner favor with outsiders (Owczarzak 2010). Granting privileged status to some but not others, inspiring competition over programs and finances, was a key tactic for countering the activist imagination in Mozambique. It resulted in compromised activists whose organizations—just like many people and governments in the developing world—barely survive. Asking for one thing, but settling for another, patients and activists got downgraded in importance. Poorly remunerated, these new paths eroded their gains, and hampered the experience of transition on the ground—from subject to citizen and back again. By the second decade of the 2000s, most activists and support groups faded politely from the scene.

In *Landscapes of Activism*, I chart such transitions at the level of ethnography and fieldwork and against the trend in anthropology to highlight globalization, the cultures of bureaucrats, and the mechanics of international aid. From the single-issue HIV/AIDS agenda, influential foundations have cut and run. Top-down projects have restrategized and rebranded. Expanding programs of medical intervention have become more broadly construed, lumping all patients—especially in the developing world—into one impotent category. Central government policies on strengthening health systems bypass local authorities, reducing needs assessment and service provision to numbers instead of meaningful encounters. Consumerism has resurfaced as a main governance strategy, replacing "rights talk" as a language upon which everyone can agree. The world was assumed to be becoming more amenable to human rights, like those originally demanded for and by AIDS activists, but instead has divested itself from causes and concerns too convicting in the name of efficiency and maximizing benefits.

Considering these predicaments, the now apparent irrelevance of Mozambican AIDS associations is hardly "natural" at all, but rather, an expected outcome. Like any other idea or product that no longer serves its purpose, such groups have been deliberately "sunsetted." As a sponsored experiment, they were permitted to lapse and terminate and are now (from the perspective of management) redundant or obsolete, ready to be replaced by something simpler or easier to control.[6]

The strange decline of AIDS activism, rather than a reflection on citizen failure or apathy, is the direct result of particular forms of state and donor intervention. To conceptualize and reframe the role of AIDS activism and advocacy in the lives of patients, the strange decline of AIDS activism is a starting point for critical inquiry rather than an explanatory end. To understand this, we turn and look, perhaps paradoxically, not to the state or to doctors or donors but to the people and their stories as embedded in history. The "lessons learned" remain relevant and must not be lost.

APPROACHING ACTIVISTS: METHODS, POSITIONALITY, AND BACKGROUND

To study AIDS activism in Mozambique, I spent fifteen months there, first in Maputo (the capital city) in 2007, then in Cabo Delgado Province (in the far north) in 2009. For the bulk of my research—the ten months I spent in Cabo Delgado—I was a student on a Fulbright grant, collecting data to write my dissertation. While this constitutes the basis for this book, my experience with HIV in Africa and HIV-positive persons began much earlier, in the year 2000. Then, treatment wasn't available for HIV in Africa, except at high prices. As a Peace Corps volunteer in Zambia and a health educator, I became intimately aware of rising prevalence rates and despair on the part of those who were dying. All we could do then was hand out condoms and tell people to be careful, which only contributed to a climate of mistrust and uncertainty. Stationed at a rural Zambian health clinic on the road to Kolwezi (a town in the Democratic Republic of Congo), there was no overt support for HIV-positive persons in my village. Many discussions were held behind closed doors, encouraging people to go for tests in the city and connecting them to others who were sympathetic, if possible.

Later, in 2004, I worked with the Centers for Disease Control and Prevention in South Africa and Botswana. Private sector companies had begun to provide free treatment for their workers. Examining the effects of this was encouraging (Reed 2005; author's master's thesis). Workers were able to adhere to what were then strict pharmaceutical regimens. For companies, the payout was evident in terms of productivity, but future patients would soon benefit as well, as arguments against antiretroviral therapy (ART) in Africa began to lose ground thanks to evidence gleaned from these corporate programs.

I returned to Zambia in 2005, serving with Peace Corps Response (formerly Crisis Corps) at a faith-based NGO near Luanshya in Copperbelt Province. The NGO, Mpatamatu Home Based Care,[7] coordinated volunteers to feed and clothe HIV patients, many of whom were dying or in need of treatment. Visiting homes, bathing people, bandaging their wounds, and playing with their children, it was frustrating to know that if those infected individuals resided in Europe or the United States, they likely would have had access to lifesaving medication. A small proportion of them did, through a partnership with the pharmaceutical giant GSK (GlaxoSmithKline) but only if their CD4 counts dropped low enough to make them symptomatic.

Several survivors of that trauma, once they recovered, joined the first HIV support group I came to know well. Called the Limbani Family, named after the first man in Mpatamatu to have knowingly died of HIV/AIDS, the group met in secret and kept no official roster. When members needed help, they worked together to get it. Sometimes it was transport to the nearest hospital or a dose or two of drugs; other times, it was money for a funeral and support for new widows and orphans. The Zambian rollout of free treatment came not long after, but there was major bureaucratic red tape around actually getting it. Patients usually needed help filling out forms, obtaining identity documents, monitoring their health, and maintaining contact with clinicians after they were enrolled.

I then went to Tanzania to work with *Médecins Sans Frontières* (Doctors without Borders, or MSF), as the health education coordinator for an HIV treatment program in Makete District, in the Southern Highlands. HIV prevalence was estimated in that area at around 40 percent (Daniel 2014), and the government was not yet providing medication. MSF provided drugs in the local hospital. The project also supported HIV-positive persons by starting a support group. Called Masupha (Makete Support for People with HIV/AIDS), the support group rented an office in the district capital, which was stocked with brochures, pamphlets, and booklets about HIV in the local language.

Masupha members, who were mostly on HIV treatment, staffed the office, keeping the doors open during business hours. People recently diagnosed as positive could drop by to discuss their results and future plans. Masupha members also accompanied us in our community outreach. MSF conducted mobile HIV testing in isolated villages. During our discussions with large crowds of villagers, Masupha members would openly share that they were HIV positive and on treatment; their stories of recovery serving as encouragement for people to get tested and discover their status. MSF tried to start other support groups in smaller villages around Makete, with Masupha's help. However, these did not thrive. The new groups rarely met, and when they did, the meetings were short, uneventful, and generally not helpful to anyone. Besides Masupha, none of them lasted very long in Makete.

By the time I met Caridade in Mozambique, I had seen numerous examples of HIV-positive support groups and knew they were important. Wondering about the sustainability and future of this phenomenon, I was interested in groups that had the least outside help but still accomplished meaningful work. One question I sought to answer was "How did HIV-positive patient groups function 'on their own?'" Another one was "How does AIDS activism manifest (if at all) in 'natural' ways in the hearts and minds of ordinary people?" I identified Caridade as one of the best groups to study with the help of AIDS activists in Maputo.

César Mufanequico, the head of the *Movimento para o Acesso ao Tratamento em Moçambique* (Mozambican Access to Treatment Movement, or MATRAM), helped me determine that civil society suffered distortions at the hands of government and some donors. Going to Cabo Delgado Province, far from the nation's capital, was one way to protect my research from some of those negative interactions. Staff from Mozambique's *Rede Nacional das Pessoas Vivendo com HIV/SIDA* (National Network of People Living with HIV/AIDS, or REN-SIDA) helped me establish contact with Caridade and vouched for my credibility. As part of my research clearance, Michigan State University's Institutional Review Board ethically approved my study. In Mozambique, I was affiliated with the *Centro de Estudos Africanos* (the Center of African Studies, or CEA) at the University of Eduardo Mondlane.

During my time in Mozambique, I administered structured interviews with seventy-five HIV/AIDS patients in thirteen different support groups or associations. The questions I asked focused on their diagnosis, how they came to be enrolled in treatment, and what kind of help they received from other patients and the group itself. I also asked about their domestic life, who shared knowledge of their illness and why, and how they coped with everyday challenges. Many became my friends and formed a kind of cohort panel. Through our work together, my frequent visits in their homes and in the offices of their civil society associations, I was able to interact with about twenty people regularly.

Keeping track of the ups and downs of their lives, we were resources for one another. I was expected to contribute, just as any friend or family member in this culture would, to the circulation of social and economic capital. They, in turn and in time, did not treat me very differently than any other member of the support group. In this way, I gained access to group meetings, as well as the many workshops, trainings, and conferences organized by NGOs, government ministries, clinic staff, and the various other AIDS associations in and around Pemba City.

I shadowed AIDS association members as they did their work, assisting new patients in the "day hospital" (HIV clinic) or teaching about HIV in schools and community centers throughout Pemba City. I documented these encounters and spoke to persons I met along the way. The Mozambican health care system relies on doctors and nurses but also *técnicos de saúde* (health technicians), who had much to say on the subject of patienthood. The *Ministério de Saúde* (MISAU, the Ministry of Health) is supported by NGO funding and encompasses HIV-specific interventions through what are called the *Núcleos*, short for *Núcleos Provinciais de Combate à Sida* (or Provincial AIDS Offices). The workers at the Núcleo were intimately familiar with AIDS association funding and politics. In Pemba, the Mozambican Network of AIDS Service Organizations (MONASO), a government-organized NGO, was particularly influential in civil society activities, including the creation, formation, and formal registration of AIDS associations.

These were some of the institutions most relevant to HIV/AIDS patients and activists in Cabo Delgado. I made regular visits to these sites—clinics, NGO, and government offices—for observational purposes and to have discussions with those directly involved with HIV care, AIDS associations, and related policy decisions. I eventually established contact with AIDS activists in other associations and support groups, visiting hospitals and civil society groups in other districts in the province and participating in programmatic activities such as home-based care, where volunteers visited the homes of patients to help them maintain their treatment regimen and contact with clinicians.

In the next chapter, I will say more about the members of Caridade and how they came together as a group. What began as a small circle of patients on treatment soon grew to be an important civil society organization intent on helping others. In a place where knowledge of the virus was scarce, Caridade spread the word that treatment really worked. I also explain more about Mozambique, as a postcolony and a developing nation, and how ART became possible in the region and in the country. An understanding of this history is important to grasp the rise and fall of Caridade, to learn from the past, and to plan for the future. Though Caridade—as a group, as well as some of its members—is no longer with us, the struggles endured and the memories made are preserved in these pages, as a warning, a salute, and, in a peculiar way, also as a celebration.

2 · "MOVEMENTS" OF THE PAST
Mozambique, Caridade,
and Treatment in Africa

You don't just pass through Pemba City, at least not in a bus or a car. It's at the end of a peninsula, which makes it something of a dead end in terms of land transportation. The airport stays busy, and the port does a good deal of trade, even though it's second to Nacala in northern Mozambique. Tourists pass through usually on their way to even better beaches on the Quirimbas Islands off the mainland coast, but other than that, Pemba City is not really "on the way" to anywhere else. Rather, if you're in the city for the kind of work I'm interested in—exploring the experiences of HIV-positive persons—chances are it's your intention to be here and not elsewhere. Pemba is not some convenient stopover for collecting data, evaluating results, and then deciding if it's a good idea to stick around. That's not to say that it's not worth a trip or that it isn't an interesting place—far from it. Instead, it is rather isolated, at least from the busyness often associated with major African highways, transport hubs, or destinations that are stopovers to other destinations. It's a good sixty kilometers even from the paved road heading farther north, making it in some ways an illogical destination for those who don't have specific reasons to get here.

That is definitely the sense I got at a restaurant in downtown Pemba, sitting across the table from Antonio, the president of Associação Caridade—a support group, or association of people living with HIV in the city. One could even say that at that time Caridade was *the* AIDS association in town—there were no others. This was in 2007, and the trend of such groups in this area was only beginning. No anthropologist had ever yet approached Caridade with the kind of request I was going to make. I made contact with the group through REN-SIDA, Mozambique's official network of people living with HIV/AIDS. Talking with them in Maputo, I had secured Antonio's phone number and was hoping to set up formal interviews with Caridade's members as an exploratory exercise to see how open the group might be to collaborating with a foreign researcher.

Antonio arrived with something of a cadre, two women who sat on either side of him, drinking Coca-Cola and looking in opposite directions at the activity going on around us at the outdoor café. People were passing by on the sidewalk carrying on their daily business, some getting money from a nearby ATM, others going into a neighboring supermarket, still others entering the Mozambique Airlines kiosk attached to the same building. Cars were swerving through round-abouts in the road up and down the hill from where the restaurant was located. I had been staying at the beach a few kilometers away, so I was still getting used to the comparatively unlazy atmosphere of the downtown area.

"So what are some of the activities of your association?" I asked him after our initial exchange of formalities. I knew very little about Caridade. I was aware that Antonio was a nurse in Pemba's day hospital, the HIV clinic, and assumed he must be more educated than many of the patients I interviewed in Maputo. He had his hands clasped on the table, and his brow was a bit furrowed, giving off a concerned and serious vibe. "Well . . . Seu Cristiano, is it?" He confirmed my name, and I nodded. "We are still new, I guess you could say, still in the process of being really recognized by most of the patients who come to the hospital. But *graças a deus* [thanks be to God], we do have funding, so some of our members are able to be activists." He was referring to a conceptual divide among association members.

"Activism," in Mozambican AIDS associations, doesn't mean thinking in a particular way about one's treatment or disease status. It has nothing to do with organizing protests or subverting the system. It doesn't even mean being trained by an NGO or the government in a particular activity, such as home-based care, or having some certificate stating that one has completed a course in the significance and meaning of human rights, for example (although those things bring someone a step closer). Activism, for those involved with the AIDS association, means having a paid position within the group. Anyone else is con-sidered a member, something akin to an activist-in-waiting because the goal for most members is to eventually see financial compensation for their involve-ment. This meant that some partner was financially and programmatically sup-porting the association because while everyone, even members, were entitled to handouts—for example, if a local NGO or church or even the hospital decided to give out free food to HIV positives—being an "activist" signified receiving a *subsídio* (a salary) in the form of *meticais*, Mozambique's currency.

"Basically," he continued, "we have three programs. Some people work in the hospital. . . ."

I interrupted, "Opening *processos*?" referring to new patient case files.

"Yes," Antonio replied, "helping new patients accept their [disease] status, talking to them about the medication, offering support. Then, some work with Medicos del Mundo." This was the Spanish-based NGO helping staff and run Pemba's day hospital, providing drugs and logistical support; it had begun to focus on activities outside of the city.

"These activists do home-based care."

"So," I asked, "visiting patients in their homes . . . ?"

"Yes, and finding those who don't return to pick up their medications, the abandoners. Then, we also have activists in the schools. They visit and talk about prevention, awareness, *esse tipo de coisa* [that kind of thing]."

"With the primary schools?" I asked.

"Yes, but some are in the secondary schools too. It's a partnership with the Ministry of Education."

"And UNICEF?" I asked.

"Yes, and UNICEF." Antonio paused. "So you know about that? That is a new one."

"Maria told me about it in Maputo," I responded. I heard about that project at RENSIDA's office. UNICEF, in fact, was the project that brought Caridade into RENSIDA to begin with. The association previously had no relationship with this UNAIDS-funded entity, whose leadership was appointed by the ruling political party.

At this point, I still had not visited Caridade's office. Earlier, on the phone, Antonio told me to meet him here because finding the office would be too difficult because I didn't know the city. I had seen the day hospital, though, the local HIV treatment center. It was a busy place, located in a building separate from the main hospital, with its own entrance on a side street but within the same compound. The waiting room was full, and people moved in and out of the doorways at a dizzyingly high turnover rate. I spoke briefly with a Mozambican health technician there who told me the Cuban doctor on staff was too occupied to stop work for a discussion. I meant to return later, hoping to track down Antonio there, but when he responded to my phone call, I didn't make it back until later in the week.

Unsure of what his response might be, I asked Antonio if I could sit down with members of his AIDS association to interview them for my research. I began to explain my project and was about to pull out my list of questions to show him when he interrupted. "I think, Cristiano, I think that's fine. We are very open to visits like this. There is no problem." He then began addressing the women in Makua, and while I was unable to follow the conversation precisely, I could tell it was about logistics. Turning his attention back to me, he asked, "When do you want to start?"

That afternoon I was escorted to Caridade's office, and Antonio crafted a schedule for me to interview a couple of people a day. I spent the next two weeks with Caridade members, mostly in a formal interview setting but also visiting people in their homes, strolling through parts of Pemba that were off the beaten path, joking, and talking about life in general. One day, I traveled with a few of them to a village called Mieze to visit a neighboring HIV support group, *Ajuda à Próxima*, which had splintered off from Caridade because of the distance from that village to Pemba City. Participation in Caridade meetings was difficult because of the twenty-kilometer distance, and this support group was seeking to get officially registered as a new AIDS association with the government. There seemed to be a rising tide of people with HIV organizing themselves into support groups. I was told about others that may be starting up.

Everywhere I went in Pemba, whether to interview NGO or government staff, go shopping in the market, or even walking on the beach, I ran into Caridade members. The group seemed integrated into the fabric of daily life in the city, the members stayed busy and were respected in the more formal institutions, like Medicos del Mundo, and in the day hospital. The kind of work they did there was as Antonio described—staying close to the new patients in the hospital, ready with advice, and frequently fetching people from their homes when they didn't show up for clinic visits, sometimes with the help of the hospital's ambulance, sometimes not.

Antonio himself was often in the back of the hospital with rubber gloves on, prepping patients for a visit with the doctor. Pemba City, in spite of the crumbling classical Portuguese architecture, seemed full of hope through the lens of Caridade members and activists who were happy to have a day hospital and proud to have NGOs and government staff interested in including them in programs and activities to help other patients and community members.

Caridade, like other Mozambican AIDS associations, owes its existence to what is now a long history of social activism for people living with HIV. The group began with fewer than fifteen people in 2005 and a little more than a year later was signing contracts with international NGOs, paying office bills, and filling out reports with data and deliverables like "number of people served" or "number of educational activities performed or carried out." While Caridade was, in some ways, a direct descendant of the PWAs groups discussed in chapter 1, in other ways, it was quite a distant relative. Many of the cultural and historical factors that contributed to its formation have as much to do with Mozambique as with HIV.

Mozambique is a nation still fraught with some of the same postcolonial tensions as neighboring southern African countries: issues of poverty, poor health care and general education, corruption, and rural-urban inequity. Other tensions more specific to Mozambique resonate with themes of slavery and liberation, imperialism and war, tradition versus modernity, communism and democracy, and attempts toward unifying a nation that has long been exploited, fought over, and forced into contested and fragile submissions.

This chapter is devoted to the confluence of factors that made Caridade's existence possible, as an HIV-positive support group and as activists unique to their part of the world. I begin with an overview of Mozambique's pre- and postcolonial history, including the North, an area often considered to be "cut off" from the more developed South. I also discuss how demands for treatment and other circumstances on the continent gave rise to African AIDS activists, including South Africa's TAC. The origin and inception of Mozambique's "day hospitals," or AIDS clinics, provides important context for how and why AIDS associations became part of the country's therapeutic landscape. Finally, I introduce more fully some of the main characters in this book, members of Caridade, highlighting my initial interactions with the group, along with the socialist "blueprint" for civil society that they inherited as citizens of Mozambique and Pemba City, in Cabo Delgado Province.

CABO DELGADO, THEN AND NOW

Cabo Delgado is a province in which important episodes in Mozambique's history unfolded. It was there that the Mueda Massacre occurred in 1960. Considered to be the unofficial start of the country's war for independence, shots were fired by the white colonial government on black Africans protesting oppression. It was there, also on the Mueda Plateau, that a clandestine Mozambican Liberation Front (Frelimo, or *Frente de Libertação de Moçambique* in Portuguese) first organized, inspired by a newly independent Tanzania and training and arming villagers-turned-guerrillas in the jungle.[1] It was in northern Mozambique that the Portuguese first landed, on Mozambique Island in Nampula Province, in 1502. What they found then was a thriving slave trade, dominated by the Islamic sultanate in Angoche (Newitt 1972a). It was also in northern Mozambique where the last active slaving in East Africa continued for twenty years beyond the World Antislavery Convention of 1840. Ironically, it was an end to slavery that broke up powerful, long-existing Shirazi[2] economic networks, finally permitting the Portuguese to penetrate farther into the mainland. Prior to that, Portuguese possession was limited to the extreme coast—Mozambique Island, Mossuril, and Ibo Island.

Along with ports in Angoche and the Tungue (present-day Palma), the Bay of Pemba—the third largest natural bay in the world—was firmly rooted along the Swahili Coast as an important foothold providing slaves from the mainland. Conditions there dictated the requirements for coordinating such a large-scale movement of people-as-merchandise in Mozambique. Loose confederacies of chieftainships collaborated with the highest bidders; this organizational strategy was necessary for at least a couple of reasons. One was that Mozambique's coastline is immense, bordering 2,500 kilometers of the Indian Ocean (nearly the length from Florida to Maine), and much of it is swampy or dotted with sandbars and coral reefs. Navigation was difficult, making it prime territory for small-time smugglers or coastal traders and discouraging of well-established, regular shipping routes. Another reason was that societies in northern Mozambique, in the interior, were fiercely independent. The Bantu migration and subsequent cultural integration and diffusion occurred over vast lands of isolated villages, dense forests, raging rivers, high plateaus, and steep escarpments—all of which discouraged larger, more sedentary, and politically unified kingdoms or settlements.

Because the hinterlands and much of the coastline functioned as a secure and natural defense against foreign penetration and given the success Muslims enjoyed in building up an anti-Portuguese front among the Makua-speaking peoples who lived there, Portuguese "occupation" was not fully achieved in northern Mozambique until 1910 (Newitt 1972b). Formally settled, Pemba was originally named Porto Amélia, after the Queen of Portugal. What surged then, replacing the trading of slaves (and some ivory), was the export of rubber and to a lesser extent cashews, various types of plant-based gums and resins, and a vibrant economy around the production of sisal fiber. This was complemented by cotton in the interior, in places like Macomia and Montepuez, for which the overland market routes determined the current layout of paved roads and infrastructure.

Cabo Delgado, today in 2017, isn't the most prosperous of the country's provinces, but it isn't the worst off either. Urban areas, including Pemba, are rapidly growing and increasingly targeted for foreign investment. Recently discovered natural gas reserves are projected to yield profits in the billions of dollars for some businesses. Tourism is booming, including U.S.$1,000 per night luxury bungalows on otherwise deserted islands. High-quality ruby gemstones were just discovered, in 2009, and are being heavily mined. Yet wealth is very unevenly spread. Only 50 percent of residents have potable water, and just 45 percent have access to a latrine, leading to frequent outbreaks of cholera (INS 2015). Just 17 percent of residents have electricity, and less than 3 percent have automobiles (compared to about 22 percent in Maputo City). Cabo Delgado, and northern Mozambique, remain "cut off" from successful development yet oddly connected to the "right" kind of extractive markets in ways that do not differ all that much from the past. Illegal trawling for fish and prawns represents millions of U.S. dollars lost for the government (Hill 2016). Rampant smuggling is ongoing for hardwood and timber, ivory, rhino horns, and even people as sex slaves, domestic workers, and unpaid, forced farm labor (U.S. Department of

State 2014). Northern Mozambique remains part of both formal and shadow economies, suggesting that the country has not fully escaped colonialism's errors and lingering effects.

MOZAMBIQUE, THE POSTCOLONY

As a Portuguese colony, Mozambique was subject to *chibalo* labor, which, even after the abolishment of slavery, enforced a plantation-like existence upon the majority of the rural population (Harris 1960). The Portuguese-run *companhias* (companies) dominated the economic landscape, turning goods produced through coerced fieldwork into economic profit for Portugal. This system eventually degenerated into full-scale anticolonial sentiment in the country, and war broke out in 1964. Nationalist unity was achieved in Frelimo, which was then a guerrilla movement but would later become the ruling party postindependence. Especially between 1970 and 1974, Frelimo successfully fended off intense counterinsurgency campaigns by stretching the air and ground resources of the Portuguese—who were fighting simultaneous revolutions in two other colonies (Angola and Guinea). Nevertheless, Mozambique's colonial war was violent and prolonged. Due to troop shortages, the Portuguese even "Africanized" their army by recruiting Mozambicans.

Such military strategies ultimately failed in Mozambique, and the nation's independence coincided with Portugal's own turn to democracy and the defeat of the dictatorial military regime there in 1974. This year marked the end of Portugal's official rule over all its colonies, and a transitional government facilitated the transfer of power from Portugal to Frelimo. As the new ruling party, Frelimo espoused Marxist ideology, seeking a socialist postcolonial order similar to the combined nationalist and revolutionary ethos of countries like Cuba, Russia, China, and Vietnam. Socialism thus became the ideological stance of Frelimo at independence, a decision that had serious impacts upon its economic development policies, especially concerning the rural areas. Centralized decision-making became standard, and Frelimo considered itself the sole representative of the Mozambican people, leaving no room for argument, challenge, or debate.

The intentions of Frelimo—and the primary way it gained credibility among Mozambicans—lay in campaigns of nation building oriented toward the modernization of society. These programs emphasized the provision of education, health, and basic services throughout the country. This began with the organization of a literacy campaign and the universalization of primary education, efforts that were intensely pursued from 1975 until 1981. Consequently, illiteracy rates dropped from 95 to 75 percent, and school enrollments doubled to 1.4 million (Chabal et al. 2002). Another effort, the "fight against hunger," instituted varying approaches to increasing production in the agricultural sector (Wardman 1985).

A similar and parallel campaign sought to bring health care to rural areas so that a clinic or regional hospital was within reach of nearly the whole population. Frelimo's modernization campaigns were envied by other decolonizing African nations, and the party viewed their progressive programs as essential to meet the population's needs and ensure its prosperity.

Due to the lack of representation and power sharing, however, Frelimo's policies were not popular with everyone. Mozambicans, particularly in the rural areas, became frustrated with the party's transformation into an intolerant structure of political control. Frelimo viewed its modernizing campaign as hinging on an accompanying reform of customary law, women's equality, and the revision of legal processes at the village level. The drive to replace traditional law and social practices failed to win widespread popular support, excluding whole categories of people from party politics, including former colonial servants, wealthier people with private incomes, assimilated ex-colonials, members of churches, polygamists, and traditional chiefs (Munslow 1986). To complicate matters, the effects of colonial war in Mozambique both legitimized violence and spread arms throughout the country, leading to a militarization of postcolonial politics. War also had numerous other negative effects, including marginalizing the Africanized forces that had fought with the Portuguese. Moreover, Frelimo was confronted with ethnic, religious, and regional polarization, particularly from the Makua-speaking people in the North.

Besides misplaced and excessive confidence in these modernization policies, the Frelimo leadership also believed it could financially and militarily support the African nationalist causes in South Africa and Rhodesia without suffering retaliatory consequences. On this point, Frelimo was very wrong. The Marxist government was vehemently opposed by Mozambique's neighbors, especially Southern Rhodesia (now Zimbabwe), which was still under the oppressive rule of Ian Smith's white, capitalist, and racist regime. The Rhodesian secret services fostered the creation of the *Resistência Nacional Moçambicana* (Renamo, or the Mozambican National Resistance), an armed guerrilla movement politically and ideologically opposed to Frelimo. Initially an external force, Renamo quickly became an internal one, capitalizing on Frelimo's inability to meet demands from rural areas and the government's unpopular, top-down programs. The civil war that ensued between these two groups became one of the most violent and bloody engagements in the history of the continent (Schafer 2001).

Renamo, therefore, sprang into existence alongside Mozambican independence, relying heavily on the ostracized white colonials and black African troops that first fought for Portugal (Vines 1991). In addition to furthering Rhodesia's aims, it also came to be a mechanism for South Africa to intimidate Mozambique into withdrawing support for the antiapartheid African National Congress (ANC). With the South African military backing Renamo, tensions grew particularly high in Mozambique between 1980 and 1983. Renamo's destructive physical attacks focused upon Frelimo's successes: the roads, railways, schools, and health centers that represented the fruits of the modernization campaigns. Renamo also carried out violent civilian massacres in the rural areas, sometimes wiping out entire villages, and recruiting child soldiers to swell its ranks.

Along with Renamo's attacks came a rapid decline in what had been hopeful gains since independence. Agricultural production slumped and some parts of the population began to flee across borders, becoming refugees in nearby countries. By 1983, Mozambique was importing 30 percent of its basic food requirements (Abrahamsson 1997). High oil costs pushed the government into a hazardous policy of fiscal borrowing. Frelimo then began to backpedal on its socialist claims and tried to separate itself from the Eastern Bloc support it had received until that point, with the aim of seeking diplomatic, military, and financial assistance from Western nations.

Backed into this corner, Mozambique joined the IMF in 1984, and the country negotiated its first debt rescheduling. It also agreed to limited peace negotiations with South Africa in the Nkomati Accord, which began a process of defunding Renamo. While a military victory was still being sought on both sides, each one initiated diplomatic tactics to establish itself as legitimate and worthy of international support. Frelimo portrayed Renamo as ruthless armed bandits who preyed on an innocent population. Renamo portrayed itself as a legitimate anticommunist movement. Firmly entrenched inside the country, Renamo found support from the peasantry, tribes, and chiefs, especially in the North, which eventually led to its formal coalescence into a political party. While Frelimo found it impossible to eliminate Renamo, Renamo also found it impossible to destroy Frelimo's political legitimacy. This led to a full-fledged peace agreement in 1992, with the involvement of the U.N. and the Vatican (Serapião 2004).

When multiparty elections were held in 1994, Frelimo won and has maintained power ever since. The impact of this drawn-out affair has been the maintenance of Frelimo's party structure, accompanied by complete reversals in its original socialist policies. This unique mixture—of a democracy being presided over by former champions of socialism—has meant that for many the promises of a successful transition to independence remain unfulfilled. The original vision of a unified class struggle has given way to the identification of poverty as a technical problem by persons in privileged positions, but the underlying implication is still such that speaking out against Frelimo can be considered reactionary, making one an unauthentic citizen or an enemy of the state (Igreja 2008). In this mode, and in partnership with diverse other nonstate actors,

Frelimo continues to dominate decision-making in government, the direction of policy, and the provision of services for the population through both direct and indirect means.

There are a number of ways in which this dominance plays out, but one odd and notable feature is the distance—both physical and cultural—between the seat of government (the capital city of Maputo) and the rest of the country, particularly the isolated districts in the North. In the same way the Frelimo government unrealistically claimed to represent the peasantry after independence, so does the government today govern from Maputo yet claim that its practices benefit the whole nation. This postcolonial situation exhibits the same type of favoritism shown toward the South by the old Portuguese government. All national government offices are in Maputo, a city with tarred roads and access to more developed South Africa and its markets. The electrical and water supply is reliable, and most businesses and offices have telephones and email access. The workers are more skilled and better educated than in other parts of the country.

In contrast, up north even the city roads are potholed, and pavement is so broken that they turn to dirt and thick sand in patchwork fashion, making travel particularly difficult in the rainy season. Goods are more expensive, and quality items from South Africa are more difficult to obtain. The isolation from Maputo in this regard is so strong that many traders in Cabo Delgado prefer to import from Tanzania than from the South. Communication is often limited to radio and, increasingly, cell phone, but email and internet are less available, negatively affecting the efficacy of the private, nonprofit, and government sectors. Evidence is mounting that the government makes all types of business in Mozambique difficult, including civil society, through excessive bureaucratic red tape.

We will see how this plays out for Caridade, and other AIDS associations, as their members try to eke out a living and secure a formal place in a malfunctioning political economy. Compared to many other southern African countries, conditions for AIDS activists in Mozambique are distinctly less favorable, leaving little room for support groups and activists to thrive on their own, without government support or approval. Yet even though ART and treatment activism arrived much later in Mozambique than in other parts of Africa, activists there were not unaware of their "rights." Nor were they willing to sit idly by, not participating or taking advantage of the wider political and medical freedoms being sought by other activists, especially in nearby South Africa.

AFRICA, ART, AND SOCIAL "MOVEMENTS"

From what we know, HIV started in Central Africa in the mid-twentieth century, the result of cross-species transmission from chimpanzees to humans (Nattrass 2007). Isolated cases of infection grew to epidemic proportions in a context of urbanization, increased international trade, and migration. Sub-Saharan Africa continues to be the epicenter of new cases. Half of these are young people, more than half are women, and two-thirds of all people living with the virus are African. Three-quarters of deaths due to AIDS are in Africa (UNAIDS 2016).

Before the advent of ART, 80 percent of those with HIV/AIDS died within two years. Now those on ART have an 80 percent chance of survival within that same time span (WHO 2013). Global AIDS deaths peaked in 2005 at 1.9 million and were less than 1 million by 2015, largely because of ART access (UNAIDS 2017). The ART scale-up has averted more than six million deaths in resource-constrained settings and given patients life expectancies similar to those of healthy people. In 2016, according to the latest figures, more than 53 percent of those in need had access to treatment. However, the benefits of ART should not be taken for granted. Getting to this point has not been easy. Moreover, treatment in Africa was not always considered desirable (by some major donors) or a viable option.

At the Vancouver International AIDS Conference in 1996, UNAIDS director Peter Piot stated that nobody can call AIDS an inevitably fatal, incurable disease anymore (Iliffe 2006). This marked a shift in views, a point in time when AIDS deaths started to become negotiable events. The therapeutic success of ART, as compared to monotherapy, resulted in an 84 percent decrease in HIV/AIDS mortality between 1997 and 2001 in Europe and North America. However, in 1996, the annual cost of such a regime lay between the prices of U.S.$10,000 and U.S.$15,000 per year per patient. ARVs made their way to Africa despite this, and private use flourished.

Self-medication and shadow market availability meant treatment anarchy in the eyes of some experts, with infected persons taking one or two pills inconsistently and dangerously mixing classes and types of drugs. Early clinical trials on the continent would later be dubbed unethical, primarily due to the controversy surrounding the use of placebo arms, when the effectiveness of AZT and Nevirapine (for the prevention of mother-to-child transmission) had already been well documented. Some sufferers (particularly South Africans) were receiving ART through private insurance and company-sponsored programs that provided medication as a cost-effective business measure (Reed 2005).

In 2000, at the Eighth International AIDS Conference in Durban, South Africa, the possibility of ART for Africans in the public sector was further debated. The World Bank, USAID, and other donors were dismissive of the idea, operating under claims that treatment was not cost effective and that only efforts to support prevention would be supported. The capability of Africans to adhere to complex medical regimens was questioned. USAID's director, Andrew Natsios, stated, "Many Africans don't know what Western time is. You have to take these drugs a certain number of hours each day, or they don't work. Many people in Africa have never seen a clock or a watch their entire lives. And if you say, one o'clock in the afternoon, they do not know what you are talking about. They know morning, they know noon, they know evening, they know the darkness at night" (Donnelly 2001: A8).

This sparked rampant criticism from activists about institutions being out of touch. There were also (what are now unfounded) concerns over the rapid potential mutation of HIV given poor drug usage patterns. African patients were considered by some as noncompliant because they were perceived as going to traditional healers, not returning for clinical appointments, and stopping treatment when they felt better. The fear of potential mutated virus strains, resistant to pharmaceutical intervention, was presented as a threat to public health in the popular press. People were implicated for being "as negligent with pills as they are with germs," spawning "drug-resistant forms of tuberculosis" (Huber 2007). Justifications for refusing treatment to potentially noncompliant patients raised concerns that drugs "wasted" on the poor would strengthen a virus. The specter of resistant HIV strains was magnified by reports that such strains were transmissible between humans, and treatment provision continued to lag in the public sector.

Research began to appear citing high adherence to treatment regimes in a wide variety of contexts, and the obvious double standard of adherence between countries in the North and the global South. A study in Cote D'Ivoire showed that adherence to follow-up in Africa could be higher than in Western settings if economic barriers, such as user fees and transportation costs, were removed (Nguyen 2007). Studies from Uganda, Zambia, and Cape Town reported adherence rates of 90 to 95 percent (Oransky 2003). The directly observed therapy model used in Haiti by Paul Farmer's organization, Partners in Health, showed that effective monitoring could work in a "buddy" system (Koenig, Léandre, and Farmer 2004). A later meta-analysis found pooled estimates of adherence in North America at 55 percent and in Africa at 70 percent (Mills et al. 2006). Eventually, experts would agree that HIV drug resistance, while extremely dangerous to the individual, is hard to avoid once treatment begins but not nearly as dangerous to public health as some other, more easily transmitted viruses, such as extremely drug-resistant tuberculosis (Kapp 2007).

Where it was tried, challenges to the successful uptake of publicly provided ART became evident. In Botswana, the first African government to initiate treatment for adults, medications expired on the shelves as patient enrollment remained low. Well-stocked clinics and modern laboratories did not translate into patient participation, and many people arrived already symptomatic. Because medical staff shortages, poor training, and social stigma posed problems, the country began collaborations with NGOs, communities, and patients in order to increase enrollment and demand. In other countries experimenting with public treatment, poor public health infrastructure posed logistical problems for disease surveillance, patient monitoring, and drug distribution. In those situations, patients living in the target areas of NGOs involved in treatment provision or organizations and companies carrying out clinical trials had better access to medication and services (Kalipeni et al. 2003).

The case for ART in Africa was also influenced by a successful rollout in Brazil, which after just a few years achieved nearly universal enrollment (Biehl 2006). Success in that nation was based on well-structured partnership plans, coordinated private and public interest, and the support of political leaders. The costs of hospital admissions and emergency services were offset by hundreds of millions of dollars in savings spent on ARVs. Strong social mobilization and civil society involvement were key elements in achieving and maintaining distribution. Efforts in Brazil led not only to manageable pharmaceutical pricing for ARVs but also to an increased market potential for fixed dose combinations. After Brazil showed potential, the Indian manufacturer Cipla began producing a three in one pill and a variety of other ARVs for Africa, and other pharmaceutical companies started offering price cuts. With these developments in feasibility, costs, patient rights, and drug formulations, treatment access in Africa became a substantial part of policy consideration, and arguments against the public provision of ART dwindled.

In this context, the concerns, objectives, and missions of the biomedical, political, and activist communities converged, and the effort to expand access to treatment was taken up by institutions and funders on a global scale. In 2000, the United Nation's Millennium Development Goal number six indicated that by 2015 the world will have halted and begun to reverse the HIV epidemic with implicit commitments to expanding ARV programs. In 2001, the virus was acknowledged as a major threat to international development during the U.N. General Assembly Special Session on HIV/AIDS (UNGASS). This commitment stressed the importance of a comprehensive response that included leadership, resources, and measurable targets for prevention, treatment, and care. Following the UNGASS declaration, at the 2001 summit of the World Trade Organization, activists succeeded in lobbying for the right to health over proposed deals for patent holders and drug manufacturers. This victory allowed for a less-harmful version of the Trade-Related Aspects of Intellectual Property Rights (TRIPS) agreement, as it impacts the importation and distribution of pharmaceuticals.

In 2002, the Global Fund to Fight AIDS, Tuberculosis, and Malaria was launched at the U.N. General Assembly Special Session on AIDS in New York City. The purpose of the Global Fund was to increase donor aid to fight these three diseases and to coordinate the resources available for them. The Bush administration, in 2003, launched PEPFAR, which eventually became the most highly funded global program with the sole aim of treating and preventing HIV worldwide. That same year, the WHO and UNAIDS started the "3 by 5 Initiative," with the aim of providing treatment for three million people by the end of 2005. While this and many of the other targets set by the programs and institutions mentioned here were not met since becoming a main component of the agendas of such institutions and programs, access to treatment has continued to improve.

The role of activism and civil society in the expansion of treatment in Africa has been important, understated, and poorly documented except for a few cases. While anthropological insight has centered on this phenomenon as a social movement and as political resistance, little is known about earlier examples on the continent that gave rise to what we now know as African AIDS activism. This is in part due to the initial proliferation of scattered groups whose existences were not well publicized or funded. One of the first might have been Zambia's Positive and Living Squad (PALS), which focused on care and advocacy and started in 1991 (Zulu 1993).

Another, which began as a collaboration among patients, government, and an NGO, came out of the Dakar hospital in Senegal, and it is in this country where the first example of an "umbrella organization" of people living with HIV appears. The Network of African People Living with HIV/AIDS, which started in 1993 and had two million members in 2005, may have been a blueprint later adopted in other nations as disparate groups came together as loose associations with representative members from different cities, districts, or provinces. Lumiere Action, started in 1994 in Abidjan by Dominique Esmail, gives us the first example of an HIV positive leader refusing to take ARVs until they were available to the general public (Lumiere Action 2015).

By the early 2000s, thousands of similar groups had sprung up across the continent, characterized by different purposes, intentions, and results. These African groups differed from the AIDS activism found in the United States, Europe, or Brazil, where the foundation for community and political action was based on homosexual identity. Activism in this part of the world was less centered on resistance, the carrying out of independent prevention campaigns, or the direct shaping of policy as enacted by the state—best described, perhaps, as "activism within the state" (Biehl 2006: 212). While wanting their demands to be heard, early activists in Africa were not primarily concerned with being antithetical to government. They were not as accustomed to stigma as gay activists and so were less likely to declare their status in public. Many early activists were also women (Iliffe 2006). Well positioned to work with NGOs and the state in dual aspects related to gender and health funding, the demography of involvement in African groups reflected not only a generalized epidemic but also the objectives of international organizations and institutions.

Examining the place of AIDS activism in the history of ART in Africa, South Africa stands out as an exception. This is due not only to the legacy of apartheid but also to the successful leveraging of international networks (Grebe 2011). Early groups established by white homosexual men, such as Body Positive (which started in 1987), later came together with black African support groups to form the National Association of People with AIDS (NAPWA, which started in 1994). NAPWA was not considered particularly grassroots in nature because of government sponsorship. When the African National Congress (ANC) took power, however, relationships between the government and activists started to break down.

The ANC refused to work with NAPWA and many other NGOs and reduced financing significantly. When the government stopped testing AZT in the country, NAPWA's refusal to contest the national AIDS policy led to the formation of a splinter group known as the Treatment Action Campaign (TAC). TAC undertook the first example of major political action by HIV-positive Africans, protesting in the streets, staging "die-ins," and blocking the entryways of government buildings in an effort to reverse the government's lack of interest in public ART provision.

Named after a section of the American organization ACT UP, TAC also focused on direct action on behalf of PWAs. The group recalled the protest tactics of the antiapartheid movement, drawing in a diversity of South Africans including the young, poor women most affected by HIV in that nation. Zackie Achmat, TAC's international face, like other African activists before him, refused to take ARVs until they were available to the public (Robins 2006). The group had 110 branches in South Africa by 2004. TAC's early supporters included the provincial government of the Western Cape, which defied the national ban on providing AZT to pregnant women.

This allowed for collaboration between Doctors without Borders (MSF) and TAC in informal settlements like Khayelitsha in Cape Town and Lusikisiki in the Eastern Cape. With MSF carrying out medical provision and TAC focused on community education and awareness, the project contributed to understandings that Africans in poor areas were capable of adherence to medication (Cohen et al. 2009). This relationship between MSF and TAC not only aided in the approval of Nevirapine in the country but also encouraged the idea of "fictive kinship" developing among people with HIV, positioning them as drawing new kinds of identities and subjectivities from a traumatic illness experience (Robins 2006).

There is now a long history of scholarship on TAC, depicting the organization as an excellent example of civil society centered on the issue of HIV/AIDS and biomedical concerns of patient health (Grebe 2011). TAC exposed the effects of HIV where treatment was unavailable, and solidarity around ART was crucial to its success. Claiming treatment as a human right, TAC also gained status as a social movement and drew on both international and informal or local networks. Because of its success, others would later try to reproduce TAC's model, which hinged on establishing alliances among a broad-based coalition. Fusing together service provision with political mobilization, the involvement of outside forces was crucial and did not appear to displace the ability of local forces to accomplish goals.

In the case of TAC, local HIV support groups interacted with more than just people from activist, donor, or NGO circles. Connections were made involving the influences of people from fields including academics, law, international development, biostatistics, grassroots development, and religion. The "treatment as human right" discourse drew on the experiences of South Africans with years of political involvement (mostly in the Marxist Workers Tendency Movement) as well as student activists and technical experts. TAC was also able to harness the authority of international agreements, such as TRIPS and the Doha Declaration,[3] which recognized the rights of nations experiencing a public health emergency to break patent laws.

Such agreements, on the part of nations and international institutions, were integral to TAC's approach. Situational demands were articulated within wider policy contexts. For example, activists pointed to the Universal Declaration of Human Rights, which states that "everyone has the right to a standard of living adequate for the health and well-being of himself [sic] and of his family, including food, clothing, housing and medical care and necessary social services" (WHO 1948). There is also the United Nations' International Covenant on Economic, Social, and Cultural Rights (ICESR), article 12, section 1, which states that "States Parties to the present Covenant recognize the right of everyone to the enjoyment of the highest attainable standard of physical and mental health" (United Nations Office of the High Commissioner for Human Rights 1966). The African Charter on Human Rights and Peoples' Rights states (article 16, section 2) that "every individual shall have the right to enjoy the best attainable state of physical and mental health" and that "States Parties to the present Charter shall take the necessary measures to protect the health of their people and to ensure that they receive medical attention when they are sick." (Organization of American Unity 1981).

While the interpretation and implementation of these agreements vary widely, calling them into action is seen as a claim on government for the specific right to treatment or provision of health services. AIDS activists positioned these agreements as social security on more than just treatment but also on issues such as safe housing, clean water and sanitation, or information and education. This has culminated in a conception of the human right to health as a package of health care and treatment services ranging from the preventive, curative, and diagnostic along with the facilities, goods, and services required to deliver them (Hayden 2012). With TAC came the understanding that the provision of public sector ART is foundational for a normal life and that countries like South Africa have the responsibility to provide these drugs because they are necessary for the exercise of other human rights.

Therefore, TAC's accomplishments represented a turning point for activism on the African continent, positioning treatment as a major concern within a wider social movement for reducing health inequalities. This broadened the available language that patients and others were able to use in bargaining for ART and health care resources. Poor ART provision, as a health inequality, brings in concepts of power, status between countries, funding gaps, and poor resource allocation because of social discrimination and political exclusion. People are then able to bargain for essential medications or the provision of quality drugs that address the priority needs of a country's population at affordable prices. It is in the concept of essential medicines and ART provision that AIDS activist and patient needs have merged most effectively with international policy and the interests of individual nations.

Patients now have life expectancies on par with healthy people but with a crucial caveat—adherence to treatment must be sustained. This is because antiretrovirals do not cure people of the virus; rather, the pills work to lower the body's viral load so that it can continue to produce CD4+ cells. These are necessary for a healthy immune system to ward off the opportunistic infections that we all regularly encounter but that disproportionately threaten the lives of those people who are immunocompromised. Drugs are broken down into different classes, and each class intervenes at different points as the virus attempts to replicate itself on the cellular level and infect additional cells. Patients do best when they ingest drugs from all three classes of antiretrovirals or one pill that contains a formulation of each drug. These are the "fixed-dose" combinations to which most Africans now have access and are taken, ideally, twice a day.

It is not always easy for patients to tell how well their body is doing on the drugs without consistent clinical contact. Being on ART is a different sort of experience than getting better from taking a round of antibiotics, for example. For one thing, the pills are not a cure. This can be difficult to explain to new patients, especially if their understanding of biomedicine is limited. Also, patients should not gauge their level of health based only on how they feel. Regular laboratory tests must be done to measure viral load and to count CD4+ levels. Side effects can make treatment a very unpleasant experience, particularly upon initiation, making people feel worse after taking the pills than they did before, with symptoms like nausea, diarrhea, dizziness, hunger, or fatigue.

With persistence, however, viral load suppression can be achieved. Patients feel better and can work again. They will even start to look better, what some call

the Lazarus effect (Walton et al. 2004), regaining weight and energy and seeing rashes, sores, and wounds disappear. Still, many people do stop treatment,
and if they don't start again, this always leads to disease relapse. There may be
some very practical reasons for this, like poor patient counseling, transportation,
or drug availability. It may also be a kind of compromise or loss of the patient's
resolve or willpower, similar to what happens to soldiers experiencing "combat fatigue" (Jones 2006). That is why standard clinical help, without catering
to the specific needs of a population and without providing forums for support
groups and other social support, is less likely to succeed. In Mozambique, the
answer to these dilemmas—and what contributed to the formation of AIDS
associations—was the day hospitals.

DAY HOSPITALS AND THE PEN PLANS IN MOZAMBIQUE

At the time when TAC was making headlines in South Africa, the Republic of
Mozambique and its international partners were just beginning to make provi-
sions for the introduction of ART into the national health system. The government issued Ministerial Diploma Number 183-A/2001 on December 18, 2001,
which regulated the process of officially introducing ARVs into the country. It
limited distribution to a couple of hospitals and formalized a request for the
involvement of other organizations because government-run clinics reached
only 30 to 40 percent of the country's total population (Kula 2008). From 2001
to 2003, fewer than one thousand patients had access to treatment, and this
treatment was available only in the two biggest cities of Maputo and Beira.

In 2003 and 2004, Doctors without Borders and the Catholic charity
Sant'Egidio became involved, expanding the model that some Cuban doctors
had adopted from their country and were implementing in a similar fashion
across Mozambique—giving ART patients their own buildings and related services, completely separate from other hospitals and other patients (Eade and
Smith 2011). This served as the blueprint for the "day hospital" system in the
country, a system of treatment units dedicated entirely to HIV-related services.
As NGOs became more and more involved with AIDS care, the day hospital
(HDD, or *hospital de dia* in Portuguese) became a privileged place for them to
carry out their work.

Not only were HDDs usually isolated from other hospitals and clinics, but
they were also comparatively better off. They typically had their own waiting
areas, consultation rooms, and hospital beds. Patients had access to their own
pharmacies, well-trained staff, and even expensive equipment unavailable in most
other clinics, like laboratory machines and ambulances dedicated specifically to
day hospital work. Initially, patients could get everything they needed at the day
hospital—a lab test, a doctor's appointment or physical exam, medications such

as ARVs or analgesics, and education on living with the virus. Videos were often shown in the waiting areas of day hospitals, and nurses or counselors had a captive audience for carrying out activities like nutritional cooking demonstrations or water sanitation techniques.

During the pilot phase of the day hospital system, from 2004 to 2005, about thirty HDDs were in operation. The number of patients on ART rose from 7,200 to 19,000. In 2006, 120 more HDDs were opened, and the number of beneficiaries reached 44,100 patients, or 10 percent more than initially planned for that year. By 2007, 211 day hospitals were seeing patients in every corner of the country, and the number of patients reached 88,211, only about 6,000 less than the total number of patients in the country estimated to be in critical need of antiretroviral therapy (Kula 2008). Though HDDs were phased out in 2009 (a contested process I discuss in detail in chapter 5), in 2016, nearly one million Mozambicans were enrolled in ART, largely as a result of the support of PEPFAR and other donors (MISAU 2016). This represents about 65 percent of the estimated number of people in need. The HDDs helped jump-start this process but were later depicted as unsustainable by the government and others who, in the name of strengthening the national health system, aimed to have them shut down, or "decentralized"—hence the protests and outrage that I will unpack later on.

At first, however, the government was immensely favorable toward the HDDs, accepting them as part of what it called the *Rede Integrada* (Integrated Network) of its national health system (MISAU 2004). This made day hospitals into points of triage within the overall hospital network, just like maternity or pediatric wards, surgical units, and blood banks. The Mozambican Ministry of Health (MISAU) included the day hospitals in their second *Plano Estratégico Nacional de Combate ao HIV/SIDA*, known as PEN II (the second National Strategic Plan to Combat HIV/AIDS). The series of PEN plans—PEN I, II, III, and IV—were the results of governmental and donor negotiations, spearheaded initially by the World Bank, that included recommendations on reducing the impact of HIV/AIDS along with specific objectives for NGO and government health care programs (Wamba and Loga 2008).

Besides the day hospitals, the PEN plans guided the involvement of governmental ministries besides MISAU—like the Ministries of Education, Youth and Sports, and Agriculture—to conform to what the World Bank and other donors termed a "multisectoral response" to the virus. The plans also oversaw the creation of additional AIDS-specific bodies, in particular, the *Conselho Nacional de Combate ao SIDA* (CNCS, or the National AIDS Council), and its provincial subsidiaries, the *Núcleos Provinciais* (referred to simply as Núcleos, or Provincial AIDS Offices). In addition, the second and third PEN plans called for the creation of civil society groups—the AIDS associations—under the purview of MONASO, a new government-run NGO that, like many AIDS associations, eventually became powerless and defunct.

Heavily funded, issued under the guidance of the World Bank, and inviting increased involvement from international institutions like UNAIDS, the PEN plans saw renewed interest in HIV programming on the part of national political leaders, and the response was in many ways raised to a bureaucratic level higher than the Ministry of Health (Harman 2007; Hanlon 2004). The justification for this, that HIV was an international development issue and a challenge to the governance of the nation, also placed the response firmly on the agenda of Frelimo. This fit in well with the government's centralized approach and projects geared toward "high modernism" (Harvey 1991).

Particularly in the short two years after the colonial war but before the civil war with Renamo (1975–1977), Frelimo sought to universalize education and health care on a national level, making Mozambique one of the first nations to adopt the WHO's recommendations on primary health care (PHC) in developing nations, in 1977. The country was considered a leader in immunization campaigns against diseases like smallpox, tetanus, and measles, with about a 90 percent coverage rate for the nation's population—a high figure almost unheard of in the region (Isaacman and Isaacman 1983). The day hospital system, likewise, was considered a modernizing project by Frelimo, at least initially. Like cancer units or children's hospitals in developed nations, specialized treatment could be provided for select populations. HIV/AIDS patients in Mozambique had their own wards, what might loosely be called "centers of excellence," bucking the common trend of the simple, impoverished care available in other health clinics.

In the real-world setting of the day hospitals, HIV support groups first began to appear. Already a privileged site for partnerships between the government, NGOs, and multinational institutions, the AIDS clinics served also to bring patients together regularly and enabled the formation of the kind of civil society called for in the country's strategic plans. Multinational institutions purport that HIV/AIDS patients are useful in the clinic. UNAIDS called on them to advocate for themselves, to assist in the delivery of services, and to mobilize communities, especially to facilitate faster treatment uptake and less program dropout (UNAIDS 2012: 36). Clinicians believed they contributed to "task-shifting" (Bemelmans et al. 2010), alleviating the burden on health care staff by counseling new patients and preventing service-related bottlenecks in overcrowded clinics. ART patients could be treatment supporters and assist with a range of clinical duties including the filling out of forms, counting patient's pills to measure adherence, and providing "directly observed therapy" for one another—the "buddy" system (Brinkhof et al. 2010; Harries et al. 2010).

A couple of HIV-positive patient groups had been around in Mozambique since before treatment was available. Kindlimuka in Maputo and Kubatana in Beira were formed in the late 1990s. However, limited to large cities, predominately with a prevention-oriented agenda, the day hospitals were the real seedbeds for the additional growth of similar groups. Treatment, and its expansion, gave them a better-defined meaning and purpose. NGOs, like Doctors without Borders, who helped nurture TAC in South Africa, pushed for the creation of more Mozambican AIDS associations. Government bodies, like Mozambique's National AIDS Council, also became supportive, under pressure to carry out "dynamic projects" (Matsinhe 2008). To make civil society "happen" according to plan, AIDS associations were a perfect fit.

Encouraged by NGO and health care staff, Mozambican AIDS associations began to form in the day hospitals. When I first arrived in 2007, there were more than a dozen of them in Maputo. Most of these were small, consisting of ten to twenty members. They had meetings at their local day hospitals and worked within the bounds of their neighborhoods. The *Hospital Militar* (Military Hospital) and the Alto Maé Clinic (run by Doctors without Borders) were two examples where small AIDS associations sprang up. Other larger groups like Kindlimuka, the country's first AIDS association, had their own offices and ran several projects for their members for income generation and for home-based care of patients on ART.

Mozambican AIDS associations, especially the ones affiliated directly with RENSIDA, operated under a state-imposed structure. They had reports to fill out and data to submit. They undertook what were called "general assemblies," where leaders including presidents, vice-presidents, secretaries, and treasurers were elected. This was the model set out for HIV/AIDS civil society in Mozambique. It was bureaucratic and formalized. Because the system lent itself better to funding, HIV patients who formed support groups—like Caridade in Pemba—often sought to become official AIDS associations, to be recognized by the state, and therefore capable of participating in state or NGO-sponsored projects.

FIRST IMPRESSIONS: GETTING TO KNOW CARIDADE

Throughout this book I draw on data from many AIDS associations, eight of them in Cabo Delgado Province. Each of them split from or rose from the midst of Caridade, the province's first AIDS association and the one with which I had the most intense and solid relationship. I present Caridade as the prototype and the default leader of these other splinter groups. Many basic traits remain the same across each group. The situations I discuss can safely be extrapolated to the national context as well, particularly for the smaller groups not operating as "flagship" examples of AIDS associations in larger cities. According to this formula, the Mozambican AIDS association is both support group and civil society, oriented toward mitigating the impacts of the virus for its members.

One of the biggest concerns for HIV-positive persons everywhere is the threat of stigma from the community and from families. As a support group, the association exists to offset the danger posed by being socially outcast and the fatalistic outlook on life that can result from that (Roberts 2008). For AIDS activists, the association is supposed to be a harbinger of human rights, to function independently from the state, and be self-sustaining (Grebe 2011; Hayden 2012). My first encounter with Caridade, in 2007, involved only a brief introduction of two weeks. During my interviews with members, I asked a series of questions about them and about the group—how it came about, its relevance in their lives, how they helped each other stay on treatment. What I found was that these dual roles—of support and activism group—were more difficult to reconcile than it might seem.

Statements made during these initial interviews echoed a theme of hope, but to varying degrees. Some people benefitted more or less than others from the work and efforts of the association. Caridade had about sixty enrolled members at the time. Antonio, the president, provided me with a list of interviewees representing a wide range of members, of various ages, genders, and lengths of affiliation. Solidly connecting members' experiences was a change from poor to good health once treatment began. The sense that there are many other people "out there," in the city but especially in rural areas, suffering the same kinds of tragedies that Caridade members did—lying in bed for months or even years completely unaware of what ailed them—was strong and provided purpose and direction to the group. There was an atmosphere of gratitude to the hospital, the government, and the NGOs, accompanied by a commitment to recruitment, equally shared by group members, paid and unpaid. Financial and other opportunities opened up through the association. Besides small salaries (ranging from U.S.$50 to U.S.$100 per month, depending on the activity), there was a communal garden, and the group was raising goats for sale. Talk of a reduction in stigma around the virus and people who live with it was common.

Several members stated that encouraging other sufferers to get tested, start treatment, and stay on it had become a personal goal for them and a responsibility:

Before, people were scared. If you were positive, it meant death. "AIDS kills," that's what the billboards [along the highways] said. Now people are opening their eyes and are thankful. They are following the path to the day hospital. Discrimination is reducing, it's not like it was before, back when people thought that you can't eat together. There are people who don't want treatment, and the association [Caridade] is charged with helping to find them. Some try to hide, but we talk to them. It has to be like this—"let's go to the hospital together"—to advance treatment. With our help, the numbers are rising. In ten years, they probably will have already cured this [virus], that's what I think. Caridade exists so that we can show our faces. Some people here that you talk to [in the association] will tell you that they don't receive anything. They do it for the love of the job. (Helena, association member)

A long time ago, people did not want to go to the hospital—*nada!* [no way!]. But we got used to hearing it on the radio. We didn't have support [funding or jobs] then, we would just go to the hospital and educate people. We sat together for so long, then we thought, "Let's make an association, as positives." We had heard that in Maputo there is an association; in Quelimane, there is an association; in Nampula, there is an association, so that's also why we're here. At first, we were just ten people. We presented ourselves to the government, and they accepted us. We first got help from the Núcleo [Provincial AIDS Council], from a Portuguese woman there. The governor's wife was like our mother, encouraging us, helping us with projects. Now discrimination has stopped, it's not a big problem, but that doesn't mean people are taking the pills. The number of people on treatment is low because everyone thinks HIV means death. They don't know that the pills can make you *bom mesmo* [very healthy]. Like me, I stayed in the bed one year, basically dead, unable to move, like this [he feigns collapsing in his chair]. We are asking for more help, to expand treatment. Things like our garden, because it helps to expand treatment. For Caridade, we can't get tired, we have to support people not to stop treatment, not to refuse to get tested. Partners [the government and NGOs] need to help us not to get tired, so that people don't abandon their treatment. (Reggie, association member)

Further conversation revealed a different conception of stigma, specifically concerning what a "reduction" in stigma was intended to achieve.

Reggie, the man just quoted, when asked if his family knew about his illness, told me, "No! They do not know. That would not help anybody." Stigma reduction and social acceptance of persons living with the virus are separated out. According to Victoria, who was a Caridade member from the beginning, "Stigma is decreasing, but I live with this as a secret, my family doesn't accept it. Our province is the last one to get this [an AIDS association]. We feel discriminated because of this. And some [in the community] say that this association is a joke, that it means nothing. So this is the kind of discrimination we are fighting against—not the virus, but our right to meet together, to discuss our illness."

Attempting to further understand the reasons Caridade existed, its purpose, and how it functioned as a source of support, members continued to identify solidarity among patients as a tangible, desirable, and valuable result:

> Caridade is the focal point for all of the other groups that are starting to appear now—in Mieze, in Montepuez, in Moçimboa—they all started here and their leaders used to come to our meetings. They are all part of Caridade. We are in these groups to share. There is no competition among us. The objective is to get together; otherwise, people have no place to talk, to learn. We formed this group to help with these necessary things—because many people died before, when they would arrive too late at the hospital. There were few of us when we started, but the government saw the advantages of working with us and began to warm up to the idea. The Núcleo gives us money to feed members, to plant in our garden, to buy goats, and sewing machines. So it is good. We get to work together, to teach children in the schools, and to give lectures in the communities. (Iolanda, association member)

Members spoke highly of the hospital, emphasizing the consistent availability of ARVs that had enabled all of them—without exception—to maintain their treatment regimen for several years without any shortage of pills. Any treatment interruptions identified among these interview participants had occurred before they were aware of how important the pills were to their health or due to logistical challenges such as being far away from the city or other hospitals. Praise for the health care staff was common. Abdul, a man who had stopped treatment several times before becoming convinced of its efficacy, noted, "In counseling [at the hospital], they tell you not to stop taking the medication and the meaning of CD4. Maybe counseling in some places is bad, but not here."

However, maintenance of life through the support group was far from perfect. Complaints centered on access to resources for daily survival, including money and food. "Partners" and other patients were targeted for criticism:

> Now we have this problem of few donors. People want to come and be members and get something for their lives. They join the association, but then they stay in the home if they don't get paid. I don't get paid. I only get a little bit of money from UNICEF for my monthly rent. When I need money for food, where will I find it? The government should find a way to get food to us. With these donors they can get medicine to people, why can't they get food to them too? I am working to teach these kids [through the UNICEF school program], so I should be getting paid just like a government worker gets paid. I should be getting paid for being HIV positive. This is my opinion. The government needs to look at this. I feel this poverty deep in my heart. How can a girl survive living in a two-room

house with a crying baby and no money? (Anna, an association member and former school teacher)

The biggest problem for members is food. Ninety percent of us are unemployed; women are abandoned by their husbands. People live without hope. It is a mentality approaching craziness. Even if you are well educated you have little chance. The donors should give us a little stipend. They trained us as activists, so they owe us that. And each donor brings their own policy. Some put us on contracts, and we have to be in the office all day, which is not always possible. Others pay small stipends only during a project, when that is over, there is no more money for that activist. I think they are scared we will use money poorly if we have extra. But that is impossible, because you need three signatures just to get the money out of the banking account. There is plenty of oversight in that regard, we can't steal it. So now each one fights for themselves. (Alberto, an association member and close friends with the group's secretary and treasurer)

The idea of being paid to be HIV positive was presented in tandem with the idea that treatment is a human right and should therefore be free for patients. Yet in the opinion of the support group members, there just wasn't enough of an effort on the part of the government and donors to make this happen. Rebekah, one of Caridade's newest members at the time of the interview, noted, "The government should pay us—it is our father, the father of us as patients. And we are poor. We know that we have human rights. This is a big topic. Treatment is a necessity and so also is a human right. It needs to be free because it costs too much. The same thing with food and a house; we should receive incentives for those things too. Our projects stop because the donors stop funding them. Our garden stopped when the Núcleo stopped funding it." When I asked more about the association's garden, it became clear it was a project that hadn't survived for very long. Produce was stolen or disappeared before most members ever saw it.

The goats, also, had disappeared. Demands from the group to the Núcleo that the government should pay for a night watchman to keep thieves from stealing goats and produce went unanswered. People stopped working on the project because there were no benefits. Members stated that without more money, and more help from donors, Caridade's chances of success were slim. If Medicos del Mundo (an NGO) leaves, Caridade would fail, was the sentiment of many HIV-positive persons in Pemba. It was common for people to report shortages not of ARVs but of other medications, such as antibiotics, ointments, and antifungal prophylaxis, which were not available not in the hospital but only in private-sector pharmacies. As Filipe, another newer member, told me, "I've never had to stop treatment, but sometimes I go without other medications, like antibiotics, for months." Another man, Patrick, said, "At times I have prescriptions for medications that are neither in the hospital or the pharmacy, they're just not anywhere." Members of the group felt powerless over the pharmaceutical access situation in Pemba, a problem that AIDS activism, in its most popular forms, was supposed to help remedy.

Talking with Caridade members and activists in these initial stages of research yielded a mixture of the expected and unexpected. Statements about working together for the good of the community were met with claims that there was not enough compensation or benefit within the association. Claims that stigma and discrimination were decreasing were met with competing statements that seropositive status was something to be kept secret. Likewise, my impressions of group solidarity began to change further when I met one of its most vocal members—Luisa. She had been at an out-of-town training during the first week of interviews but would later become one of my main contacts in the group.

In the beginning, Luisa seemed to epitomize the prototypical HIV positive human rights activist. When I first met her for an interview, she arrived in a Medicos del Mundo hat—she worked as a home-based care volunteer for the NGO—wearing a T-shirt with the slogan "HIV Positive" written in large letters across the front. Luisa explained to me how the founders of Caridade—those who had been members since its inception, in 2004—were "stuck in their ways, old in years, and afraid to live openly with the virus." They were often demanding of or oppressive toward newer members, like her. She accused other members of being greedy. "There are some people who just want money," she said, blaming this problem on the donors. "Before the donors came, we talked to each other, after that [the group] just fell apart. Funds create problems," she told me during our first interview, looking determined and stern.

Her awareness of human rights differed from some of the other members I interviewed. Without claiming that she had the right to a stipend or a free house, her interview answers to my human rights questions were textbook material. "The government is very corrupt," she told me. For Luisa, human rights meant countering the effects of this on people living with HIV by attending government meetings and speaking out on behalf of those who otherwise wouldn't in order to maintain the current momentum toward treatment access and equality for poor, underrepresented people. This attitude was in stark contrast to the impressions I had thus far gotten from Caridade members about the meaning of human rights.

Luisa made her colleagues appear unsophisticated. I had previously been told by one man that "the government brings money for us to survive, so we like the kinds of business they do here in the city. Human rights are for me to treat my own things, like my house, or putting things in my *barraca* [his personal convenience] or the government to feed my children. This is human rights." Others suggested that they had the human right to a cell phone. Luisa's "subjectivity"—critical of the government, moving around the city without hiding her HIV-positive status—reminded me of interviews I had done with Maputo-based activists, those who were more in touch with international activists and who attended a wide variety of NGO trainings.

Luisa confided in me that she had been unjustly treated by her husband, a man from the Tanzanian island of Zanzibar, who, after having a daughter with Luisa, had kicked her out of his home, forcing her return to Pemba. She lamented being away from her only child. "Caridade is my family now," she told me, and began listing the names of others in the group who she considered her adopted brothers and sisters. Luisa had joined the association only a year ago but already seemed more involved than some of the original members. It seemed to me like Luisa would make a great partner in my research; she was forthcoming, approachable, and conformed to an idea that I had about "proper" AIDS activists—that they are politically savvy and outspoken. When she invited me to her home for dinner, I accepted. But when I suggested that we include Caridade's president, she told me, "You know, he's on his way out." She made a fist, put up her thumb, placed it against her lips, and took a swig from the fake beer bottle that her hand had formed. This was my first clue that Antonio had a drinking problem. Still, regardless of Luisa's objections, we made plans to buy some shrimp and crab from the local fishermen, and I invited Antonio to dine with us.

The next day for dinner, Antonio arrived on his motorcycle and, as I could tell from his breath and handshake, he was already inebriated. As we sat outside in the shade, Luisa and her sister cooked. Antonio told me how badly both of these women "desired" him (sexually). Luisa overheard him, gave me a quick wink, then sighed and looked away. "As the president of the association," he said, "all of these women [in the group] want me." Luisa's uncle, an elderly man who joined us for this occasion, seemed very amused with Antonio's discussion, smiling and laughing at his words and behavior. The kinds of statements the president was making must have been typical and expected.

"You know," continued Antonio, "Seu Cristiano . . . we are very poor here. We don't have anything. I don't even have enough petrol to get home on my motorcycle." At this, I became better acquainted with what Mozambicans refer to as a *pedido*—a polite version of begging, particularly targeting someone who is perceived of as having more power, resources, or money than the beggar. To *pedir*, in Portuguese, means "to ask." A *pedido* is the event or act of asking for something either in person or on paper; it is a frequent feature of social relations in Mozambique. This was often tempered with suggestions that some related favor has been or will be done—so justifying the request.

A *pedido* is formalized and summarized in the common statement, "*estou a pedir . . . dinheiro*," or "*estou a pedir . . . um cigarro*" (lit. I am asking for money or I am asking for a cigarette). Antonio's *pedido* for petrol for his motorcycle could not go unanswered on my part—a yes or no was required. The quandary in which this put me was concerning because as Caridade's president, Antonio had some power to impact my future research with the association; by refusing his *pedido*, I risked my relationship and good standing with the group. Antonio continued to drink, pulling sips from a small bottle of clear liquid that he kept in his trouser pocket. A couple of times through the evening, as we were eating outside, he fell going up and down the stairs into Luisa's home. I was hesitant to, in any way, enable this man to drive home on a motorcycle. At the end of the evening, I offered to pay for a taxi but he refused. I ended up conceding, giving him money for fuel, and he left in the dark on his motorcycle with a busted headlight. Knowing Antonio as I do now, it is highly unlikely that the money I gave him went on petrol but rather to more rounds of *nipa*, the moonshine he liked to drink.

Luisa and I became well acquainted that evening, discussing our lives and dreams with each other. I learned that Caridade would hold a general assembly later that year, and she had hopes to win the presidency from Antonio. I told her my intentions to return to Mozambique for a longer stay and agreed that I would make Caridade a part of the research. She told me more about the battle within Caridade between its founders (like Antonio and a few of the activists I had interviewed) and its *novos membros* (the new members), some of whom I had already gotten to know. According to Luisa, the concerted effort on the part of the founders to keep new members from climbing the hierarchy within the association could only fail. She told me that the new members had more education, were more committed, and would not stay *sentado* (sitting around) in their homes waiting for free handouts from the government. The NGOs that Caridade worked with knew this, Luisa said, and slowly but surely the old would give way to the new.

My initial encounter with this AIDS association yielded several conclusions. Among these, there was the idea that presenting oneself at the hospital and taking pills regularly was not such an easy thing to do. New and undiscovered patients needed active encouragement from other patients in order to start treatment. In addition, the number of those on treatment was steadily increasing. Association members felt responsible for that and proud of the ways they had helped. Also, other associations were being formed and Caridade's influence was visible. Hence there was some type of organic growth of these groups occurring, and a place for them was being carved out with more formal institutions—NGOs and the Provincial AIDS Office (the Núcleo). Caridade had a number of partners to work with, and the types of jobs activists were undertaking varied considerably. What began in the hospital among a small group of people had expanded into neighborhoods and schools.

However, the picture that was painted for me remained in many ways unverified. A brief visit with Caridade would not have been enough to know the truth. Professed humanitarian motivations—wanting to help others get on treatment, wanting to help the community—were tainted by claims of personal vulnerability, making the association, for some, a type of welfare network. Claims of selflessness, combined with notions of unrealized donor responsibility, seemed to warrant further investigation in light of the understanding that "help" seems to always come in the form of funding or money rather than from within the group itself. Projects, such as the community garden, were presented as happening and yet had already failed, and so caution had to be exercised before ascribing either revolutionary or sustainable potential to them on my part. While I had heard of the camaraderie among association members, their sincere hopes for success, and history of helping one another, the formal interview setting and the fact that my trip was quick meant I had yet to witness how well, or poorly, the association truly functioned.

In contrast with the associations whose members I had interviewed in Maputo and associated with MATRAM, Caridade had a striking number of concurrent projects. This had several implications. For example, the group had more than one boss. With plans, budgets, meetings, and activities dedicated to such disparate interests—the hospital and government, the NGO, and REN-SIDA and UNICEF (a project that also included the Ministry of Education as co-coordinator)—who is answerable for what and when can become a bit of a mess. I would later find out that these relationships were only the beginning of understanding the complete picture. Three other NGOs regularly sought out partnerships with Caridade. One was Action Aid/Pemba, which paid for the office space and other logistical infrastructure such as the two computers the group had. This NGO also sponsored short-term activities in the community, hiring Caridade members to speak at community meetings and gatherings. This project was called "Stepping Stones." It was intended to diminish stigma by having HIV-positive persons tell their stories to educate local leaders on what it was like to live with HIV.

MONASO also regularly included Caridade in public presentations. As a government-organized NGO in support of AIDS civil society, MONASO would regularly pick up Caridade members and take them to villages or schools to participate in meetings, carry out drama skits and theatre, or speak on the behalf of HIV-positive persons. Then there was FOCADE, a branch of the national LINK Forum of NGOs. FOCADE worked with Action Aid to ensure that Caridade—and other associations in Cabo Delgado—remained relevant and legitimate. They demanded reports and data from Caridade regularly, attendance at their meetings, and sponsored trainings where members would be sent to other towns and provinces to participate in skills transfer seminars, called *trocas-de-experiências* (information exchanges), with other AIDS associations in Mozambique.

This level of apparent sophistication could mean, hypothetically, multiple realities, and I knew I would have to spend more time with Caridade to figure them out. Either member claims that donors don't support the association enough were false ones or the donors were taking advantage of the members and activists by requiring them to spend their time in various activities for which they weren't well compensated. If neither of these were true, then additional explanations on the part of Caridade leaders would be necessary as to why only certain members had jobs or opportunities and others didn't. In any case, it was apparent that the abstract concept of activism may have taken a back seat to one of commerce—but this was difficult to tell because members expressed an interest in both. Certainly, from what I had seen of the multiple and small AIDS associations scattered throughout Maputo and essentially unfunded, the understanding of Pemba's AIDS activists that their province was somehow behind in progress seemed unjustified.

The coordinator of the MATRAM in Maputo once told me, "We recommend that an AIDS association do one thing only but do it very well." But Caridade was doing many things, almost anything they could, to get project funding. One realization from this initial research with Caridade was an awareness that this group was not quite capable of funding itself. Caridade members did not write grants, apply for projects, or compete for funding opportunities based on the association's own merit. Instead, Caridade looked to other organizations and groups capable of providing the resources it didn't have, and those organizations that needed a community partner looked to Caridade. The group was not generally antagonistic or critical toward the government, and so Caridade may not have been as independent as the concept of a free civil society might indicate. Like President António asking for fuel for his motorcycle, the group may, as well, thrive on the concept of the *pedido*.

AIDS ASSOCIATIONS, SOCIALIST LEGACIES

AIDS associations are not the only civil society associations in Mozambique. There are many other kinds—associations of women, schoolteachers, religious adherents and leaders, retired military, and young persons. Upon independence, the Frelimo government derived many of its political practices from the Russian revolution. The ideal was for the political party to become a ubiquitous presence and, like the Political Commissar in Russia, for a party member to be present in all activities in order to ensure the proper (nonrevolutionary) orientation of any particular group. To this end, Frelimo activists were installed in the towns and villages of Mozambique. These were the *Grupos Dinamizadores* (Dynamic Groups), party-affiliated "community" groups, composed of Frelimo enthusiasts and given objectives like organizing the collection of taxes, policing the streets, or promoting health and hygiene in their neighborhoods. Representatives were sent into all areas of the country and forcefully integrated into all working environments—supervising surgeons in hospitals, monitoring teachers in classrooms, introducing party politics to soldiers.

At the core of this, one of Frelimo's many modernization projects was party control and imposition from the top down. Some branches of the Frelimo party that still exist today got their start in this manner, with the same function now as in the past, of communicating the party's intentions or desires and educating the populations they serve—such as the *Organização da Mulher Moçambicana* (OMM, or the Organization of Mozambican Women), the *Organização da Juventude Moçambicanos* (OJM, or the Organization of Mozambican Youth), and the *Organização dos Trabalhadores Moçambicanos* (OTM, or the Organization of Mozambican Workers). Drawing on this socialist model, Frelimo embraced a marriage between nation building, community intervention, and socioeconomic change, but with the political party as the leading force, over and above the individual and even the state itself. Many of Frelimo's policies were unpopular, which is part of what had contributed to the twenty-year-long civil war.

At independence, the primary industry in the country, agriculture, was like all others, state chaperoned as well. There were state-run farms, with inputs like tractors, seed, fertilizer, and pesticides paid for by the government. Many were located on the same large plots of land where colonial farms, using *chibalo* (slave labor) from indigenous Mozambicans, were owned and operated. Then, there were farming cooperatives—the closest the government ever came to a national system of communal labor—composed of volunteer workers who shared farming equipment and implements to work large shares of government provided land. What they produced was the property of the state.

The farming cooperatives were dubbed a "movement" (similar to AIDS activism; Wardman 1985), bound together by what the government termed *cooperativismo*, literally meaning "cooperationism" (O'Laughlin 2009). Salaries were paid to members of the cooperatives, who also had access to literacy classes, shops, bakeries, and projects like brickmaking for them to build their own personal economies and homes. The Cooperative Law of 1979 stated that each cooperative should have a constitution, which set out the roles, obligations, and functions of its members. Just like AIDS associations, farming cooperatives had general assemblies and members could run for governing positions.

As noted by Wardman (1985), a defining feature of the farming cooperatives was that members demanded access to group benefits but only rarely fulfilled work obligations. Organized into "brigades," those in charge were hesitant to carry out sanctions against family members and friends or to mark those who did not show up to work as absent. Many worked just a few hours a month but got paid as if they were full time. Mobilizing people for important work proved difficult, and the organization of the cooperatives was poor. Compared to crops on private, individual plots of land, the cooperative farms were not as well watered or weeded and were not harvested at appropriate times.

Plans made within the cooperatives were often left unaccomplished. There was an obsession with bookkeeping, with registering the transfer of money, sales, and debts, but these entries were often inaccurate. Harvests rarely produced a profit. Workers had no significant incentives, and the character of the president often determined the success of the cooperative. Frelimo possessed a paternalistic attitude toward them and provided more assistance to pilot or flagship cooperatives closer to towns with greater traffic and economic activity in order to show the success of the system. People tended to care much better for their own private farms than they did the cooperatives. Producing for others and for the state did not seem to motivate people to participate for the benefit of the group and its farm.

Thirty years on, Wardman's observations appear prophetic. They point to the dysfunction of state-sanctioned solidarity and the challenges of implementing a standardized system oriented toward the organization of workers, especially at community and village levels. To include the nation and its people in radical, transformative plans, notes Pitcher (2008: 77), positions the Frelimo state as a miniature God (a "demiurge") over some of the most basic material concerns. Moreover, the focus on big projects, valued symbolically more than practically, allowed all parties to turn a blind eye to poor oversight. Plans were centralized, but mismanagement accountability was not, and so there seemed to be no one to blame when things fell apart. The AIDS associations would not escape a similar fate. Seeking and claiming insertion in state and also international endeavors seems to carry great potential for adverse effects.

There are many parallels between the farming cooperatives of the past and the various Mozambican associations of today. It is even safe to link the AIDS associations more to the farming cooperatives of socialist Mozambique than to the AIDS activist groups in neighboring postcolonial countries. Some of these parallels include a reliance on external inputs—donors, now, as well as the state—and on the driving personalities of leaders such as the presidents. The emphasis also on projects, such as prevention education, public or hospital lectures, home-based care, or the distribution of medications or products to sick people, suggests that AIDS associations must be "productive," fulfilling a specific role for the state.

AIDS associations in the larger cities or towns—flagship projects for their partners—received the most attention, visits from foreign dignitaries or program coordinators in order to make a good impression. Representatives of these associations had seats at the figurative tables of decision-making, at the donor-sponsored meetings in Maputo and at trainings abroad, as community representatives, stand-ins for the nation's population of seropositive persons. The associations that participated in this, and tow the party line—like Kindlimuka in Maputo—were "selected in" to this process. Those that didn't, like MATRAM, the Mozambican Access to Treatment Movement (Høg 2006), whose only project is holding the government accountable for treatment provision, were "selected out," barely known by the donors and multinational institutions because of their poor visibility at governmental functions.

Like Mozambican citizens just after the country's independence, through their associations, HIV-positive patient-activists came under the influence of similar types of *grupos dinamizadores*, state-supported community interventionists that emphasize and insert the ruling party's ethos into everyday life. These include RENSIDA (the National Network of People Living with HIV/ AIDS) and MONASO (the government-organized NGO overseeing AIDS civil society). AIDS associations were expected to strive for and conform to a national system of *associativismo* (O'Laughlin 2009), literally "associationism," encouraging them to band together around a cause—in this case, the empowerment of patients, or AIDS activism, for the better functioning of health care efforts on the part of the state and its partners. Experts and trainers on how *associativismo* should work in the country were sent to educate AIDS associations on how to relate to one another and how to lobby the state for their needs. NGOs were asked to participate by offering patient groups projects, salaries, and benefits.

These influences have the effect of shaping AIDS civil society, absorbing it, and reissuing it back into society after it conforms to a specific (powerless) standard. Like the farming cooperatives before them, there was deference to this paternalism—a lack of local-level motivation—leading to absolution of responsibility such that projects did not produce as they should. Patients took what they could get and did not complain. They had little vested in the venture because what bound them was not so much their illness as allegiance to an external power, one that appealed to the building of their own personal economies rather than to the moral economy or success of the group itself. *Associativismo*, as we will see, put AIDS activism on the fast track to obsolescence, making it a tool of state interests and appealing to the desires of opportunists and careerists.

3 · AIDS ASSOCIATIONS IN CABO DELGADO PROVINCE

In this chapter, I focus on the AIDS association as an institution by delving further into the everyday life of Caridade. I will describe and analyze some meetings, trainings, and encounters that occurred to the group, using these data to highlight certain findings about civil society in Pemba City. I contest understandings that civil society groups are united, that its members act in solidarity, and that the group can be independent of prevailing structures and ideologies. While AIDS associations form part of the city's "therapeutic landscape" (Gesler 1992), they are, through involvement with particular development or health projects, drawn into an organizational culture that parallels that of the state and its partners—what DiMaggio and Powell (1983: 147) call "institutional isomorphism."

While such groups should be free to pursue advocacy, social support, and political expression for people living with HIV in the area, their usefulness to a variety of actors can limit organic growth. Efforts by donors, decision-makers, and internal "leaders" to capacitate the group led to conflicts, arguments, and fission. External interference—efforts to "help" the group—might be welcome if it wasn't as inappropriate, superficial, or misplaced as it seems. Instead of contributing to or empowering HIV-positive persons in the city, the group's involvement in projects and politics often leads to what I will call "civil society existentialism." Expected to "run" itself but also to respond and conform to assistance from others, the group and its donors both become disenchanted. Yet they all continue on the same path—toward bureaucracy and economic goal setting—expecting different yet better results from preconfigured formulas, which link political progress, practical forms of activism, and international development in ways that hinder the full potential of each.

OF OFFICES AND ORGANOGRAMS

Arriving back in Pemba and becoming reacquainted with Caridade in 2009, almost two years after my first visit, I discovered that Luisa had lost her bid for the presidency. Antonio, the day hospital nurse who helped found the group, won a second term in office. I was a bit surprised to hear that. "At first, we tied," Luisa told me. "Wow, did he cry. Everybody felt very sorry for him. When the votes were recast, he won by one vote."

"So you are the vice-president now?" I asked her.

"I am the vice-president," she replied, "but we will have another *assembleia* [election] this year, and there is a two-term limit. So he has to step down." Luisa told me that everything was going well for Caridade, that the projects were continuing to develop and partners continued to fund the group.

I knew, however, from conversations I had with activists in Maputo, that funding for civil society groups like Caridade was diminishing. The coordinator of MATRAM, César, also told me that day hospitals were closing across the country, creating problems for treatment access. Soon there would be no day hospitals—this is one important place where activists had jobs and could carry out their work. Patients were also affected. "Some have already stopped coming for treatment," said César, referring to clinics in Maputo. So far, Pemba had been spared. Nobody was certain when the day hospital in Pemba would close.

Caridade's office isn't easy to find. It is surrounded by a tall, white-washed cement brick wall with the words *Latrinas Melhoradas* (VIP Latrines) painted on the outside. It is housed in the same compound as a state-run initiative designed to help city residents upgrade their outhouses with concrete floors, asbestos roofing, and deeper pits. The entrance is a large solid metal gate. After entering through it, immediately on the left, there are three model latrines, demonstrating the handiwork of the *Latrinas Melhoradas* project. At the back rests a fleet of broken-down vehicles—some lorries and military jeeps. A businessman pays the government to house them here so that he can use them for spare parts. In the late afternoon, after Caridade closes its office, the compound also hosts literacy classes for adults, an educational initiative to make up for internal displacement and scholastic face time lost during the civil war. To the right is the single-story, tin-roofed facility in which Caridade rents two rooms, one for members and another for management. There is a cement patio, well shaded by trees, just outside of the door for members. Nailed to it is the only indication that an AIDS association operates here—a piece of construction paper with the words "Associação Caridade" (Caridade Association) in wide-tipped black marker.

Inside, there is a telephone that works intermittently, depending on whether the bill has been paid. On the desk is an old computer that doesn't work. It's a monitor, a keyboard, and a metal shell: the last man who came to repair it stole all the parts inside but sent a bill to Action Aid, the NGO who pays the rent and utilities for the office, as if he had actually fixed it. There's a trash can in the corner with Action Aid's name on it but no other indication of the NGO's involvement. Taped to the walls are HIV awareness posters and ads for condoms. One features an oversized, smiling cartoon condom handing out smaller versions of itself to teenagers on a soccer pitch. On a table in the corner there is a shoebox with a slit on the top, always empty, where members can insert money to pay for *cotas e joias* (membership dues and fees). There are a couple of wooden benches and a few plastic chairs around. Carlitos, Caridade's spokesperson and my research assistant, brings them out onto the patio when he opens up the office in the morning.

There, under the shade of palm and papaya trees, members and visitors are received, usually first by Carlitos. The other room, the one for management, is usually locked. That's where the money for salaries and project expenses is kept, as are two working computers—one for balancing the budget and the other for entering data and writing reports. Bakari, the accountant, and Fevereiro, the group's secretary, spend the most time at their desks in this room. There are some books and training materials on a shelf in the corner, a couple more posters on the walls, another bench, and a reed mat. The group sometimes hosts small trainings or meetings in here if the weather is inclement.

Caridade's office, in the Latrinas Melhoradas compound, is nestled in the center of bustling *Bairro Natite* (the neighborhood of Natite), close to downtown Pemba and not far from a small health clinic and a Ministry of Health training center. It's often relatively quiet. But in spite of how cozy one might feel seated on Caridade's patio discussing Mozambican politics or some such topic, the noise just over the wall can occasionally be deafening. It rises and falls in relation to the volume and speed of motorized traffic passing by on the road outside and according to the level of music blasting from the *barracas* (small stores) just across from the entrance gate. The road is only wide enough for one car, or two motorcycles and some pedestrians. The latter have to dart out of the way whenever a car horn sounds or risk getting struck, as visibility along the winding network of unpaved roads is poor. The road is mostly sand, but that doesn't keep small rivers from forming on it and running downhill toward the ocean (a kilometer away) in the rainy season, crafting pitchfork-shaped ravines and making the paths difficult to navigate and unpredictably uneven from day to day.

A lot of what seem like small and disconnected events occur in Pemba's *bairros*, which teem and vibrate with life. Foot traffic is heavy in Natite because it is on the way to Pemba's largest open-air market, Banguia. But this bairro and places like it are more than just crossroads, to be quickly passed through. It's easy to get pleasantly trapped here and a privilege, really, to be able to stop and "hang out." With all the bamboo fences and concrete walls one might get the impression that privacy is respected, but that's something of an assumption. A lot of visiting, a lot of *bate-papo* (casual conversation) goes on behind these walls. Walking or driving along, there are gaps or cracks, and you can usually catch a peek through to the other side, into people's homes and yards.

People stop and *do* things around here. It's a thriving community rather than a simple thoroughfare. The houses and businesses—barber shops, bike and motorcycle repair huts, women roasting snack food and selling homemade brew on the street corners—represent networks and destinations in people's lives. Some people know that Caridade's office is located here—those for whom it's on their list of places to go. Others, unsure but seeking, find their way to the association in what Mozambicans refer to as *qualqueir maneira* (in whatever way)— asking around, being brought or referred by a friend. But there is no publicity about Caridade, no signs or advertisements indicating its existence or purpose to the outside world.

The office compound functioned very much like a drop-in center for the association's members and their neighbors and friends—something like a social club but with pamphlets and booklets on HIV. A steady stream of people was always visiting and found conversing on the patio. Conversation topics did not always have to do with the virus. Most centered on other aspects of survival and life in the city and the province. Women arrived and discussed their home life, including arguments with husbands and boyfriends. Men talked about their wives, children, and girlfriends or how a particular job search was going. Complaints about the government, NGOs, or certain people working with the association were common.

Caridade's office, in many ways, was a valid part of Pemba's "therapeutic landscape" (Gesler 1992; Bell et al. 1999). As an in-between place, not the clinic but not the home either, it served as another "sphere of the life world" (Kearns and Collins 2000) for members to sustain their personhood. While Pemba's day hospital was certainly a part of people's medical lives, the office served as a site for addressing other, more mundane, and less formal topics related to living with HIV in Pemba City. It formed part of what Parr and Davidson call "lived geographies" (2009: 263), a place where people found inspiration and developed coping mechanisms in their own small, personal, and transitory "niches" of survival.

On my first full day with the group, after my return from the States, I was in Caridade's office when a Landcruiser stopped and a couple of doors slammed shut on the other side of the wall. Luisa and the others had just said good-bye to Ana, from MONASO, the state-run NGO, who had stopped by under the premise of learning more about the association's action plan for the next year. During that brief meeting, she prepared the group for what should have been a surprise visit from Pemba's newest, wealthiest, and most influential NGO, the PEPFAR-funded Elizabeth Glazer Pediatric AIDS Foundation (EGPAF). It's common practice in Pemba for people to give others notice when something either promising or threatening is looming. Ana's visit should have been sufficient preparation for the upcoming encounter, but it wasn't. EGPAF was seeking a suitable community-level partner to continue, and even expand, a home-based care program in the city. Another association was being considered—Bem Vindo, which had splintered off from Caridade a few months back—and this visit was intended to clarify which one had the capacity to do the work.

As the representatives of EGPAF and Caridade sat down to talk about the association's achievements, Luisa told them about the UNICEF-funded school project that the association was conducting. It had expanded into other districts, making Caridade a province-wide association. The EGPAF workers listened to her summary and then proceeded to ask a series of routine questions, focusing on the association's demographics, budget, and number of people served through its projects. One of them then presented an organogram in the shape of a pyramid. Showing this to the Caridade as an example, it had at the top a fictional president. One level below were the positions of vice-president and president of the assembly. Other positions, including the secretary, treasurer, vice-secretary, and vice-treasurer occupied lower levels on the pyramid. Members formed a generic base block at the bottom. EGPAF asked Caridade to provide its organogram. Could they have a copy for their files? Where was the association's president—this man, Antonio—and could they speak with him?

The reactions of Luisa and the others consisted mostly of nervous glances and a brief period of silence. Falume, the president of the assembly, walked over to another area with a couple of members and began to talk quietly in a kind of huddle. "For us," responded Luisa to EGPAF, "the president is in the middle." She pointed to the center of the paper. Looking at the organogram, she said, "We don't have one of these yet." She began drawing a makeshift version of the association's hierarchical structure on a blank sheet of paper. As the EGPAF staff watched her, some brows furrowed. "This isn't possible," replied one. Luisa had drawn the chart with the president and the members in the middle, with all other elected positions in a circle around them, and no lines connecting to the president. It was explained that he wasn't there to talk because he was a nurse in the day hospital and was currently at work. In reality, he was at or near his home, drunk.

The air was palpable with tension as the association realized that the absence of a president and the lack of an organogram were two strikes against them at the outset. The conversation—what really amounted to an interview—continued but changed slightly to the form of an audit. Fevereiro was asked to produce the reports of activists and examples of documents turned in to UNICEF and Action Aid. Bakari was asked to produce printouts of the budget from the past few months, receipts from purchases, and bank account statements. At this point, questions became more specific. Why are some reports completely filled out, and others are not? Why are there no minutes from the group's meeting last January? At these targeted inquiries, Luisa appeared visibly angry. Her answers became curt, and it seemed she would be happy to just walk away from the scene.

That's what a few Caridade members did, including Falume and Carlitos, who I saw stroll out of the gate and onto the street. As the questions continued and they didn't return, I too went out of the compound to see what was going on. I found them at the *barraca* across the road—a bar-like structure complete with stools for clients on the outside—talking to the owner and drinking bottled beers that he kept out of sight for them behind the bar, just so nobody would notice. He would hand them over when the two of them requested so that they could take quick sips before returning the bottles to their hiding places. Falume began complaining to me about the meeting. "These people are not serious," he told me. "They're just trying to catch us in a lie." Carlitos told me what he thought as well. "They already have all of this information," he said. "They can get it from Action Aid or from FOCADE or MONASO or Medicos del Mundo [all partners and donors of the group]. This is more of a formality for them to be able to tell us no."

While their responses might seem immature—Luisa's impatience, the president's absence, leaders like Falume and Carlitos abandoning the discussion—their reactions might also qualify as an act of resistance to what DiMaggio and Powell (1983: 150) call "coercive isomorphism." This refers to the formal pressure placed on less powerful groups by more powerful ones so that they adopt the same structures as other "units" similar to them in purpose or function. In this encounter between donor and local group, the implication was that a contract and related financial graces could be provided if the group conforms to outside expectations. Whether the structure proposed and suggested—the organogram, with its theoretical hierarchical pyramid—was appropriate for the group or not, Caridade's inability to produce anything like it was seen as an indictment of their willingness to cooperate. It meant the group did not meet the same expectations as others and perhaps could not be trusted. I imagined that if Caridade did not conform to this specific programmatic regularity, it might not conform to others either, and I promised myself to keep watching out for that. What I realized during this encounter, however, was that this sort of direct imposition was intended to force the group to conform or risk losing funding.

Groups like Caridade can become standardized and less diverse in less "coercive" ways as well. One way is through "normative pressure" (DiMaggio and Powell 1983: 152). This refers to how socially embedded mechanisms—education, professionalization, and political influence—dominate and define the accepted methods and conditions of particular lines of work. When "normative pressures" are at play, those groups with better visibility, more wealth, donors, projects, and partners hold significant sway over the development and evolution of others, who are under pressure to conform in order to meet with equal success. Normative pressure is the realm of careerists. Those with more impressive titles, name recognition, branding, or marketing tactics attract more attention and generate more work. "Selected in" to a particular industry—like AIDS activism—the structure of the group and its techniques for problem solving become the accepted standard. For other groups to deviate from this is risky because alternative methods are not believed to be effective.

What this means for Mozambican AIDS associations is that the drive and motivation to become involved with NGO or government projects is generally viewed as healthy and helpful to the group. But this can be divisive, inspiring allegiances outside of the group itself, and it can create an environment positioning the group as a resource for opportunists. What we will see is that in Pemba, where wealth and opportunity are scarce, normative pressures influence the group to orient itself more toward benefits or commerce than to unity, handicapping its ability to adjudicate or moderate internal conflict.

REPUTATIONS: MEETINGS, CONFLICT, AND SLANDER

As it turned out, Caridade would not be awarded EGPAF's home-based care contract. The new association, Bem Vindo, would be the recipient. As other AIDS associations sprang up with whom they could work, international NGOs in Pemba were beginning to cut ties with Caridade. The group was not perceived as very hardworking. The coordinator of Medicos del Mundo, the NGO that had helped fund the startup and had initially worked closely with Caridade, had, just a couple of years ago, encouraged me to come back and study the AIDS association. Now I was being told that it had irresolvable internal problems and that I shouldn't work with them at all. "There are certain members who we believe are crooks," he told me. The NGO had even banned some Caridade activists from attending their trainings and funded the startup of the new association, Bem Vindo, to work in their community service projects as an alternative. The head of MONASO blamed Caridade's downfall on project funding. He had seen it before with associations in other provinces and told me that "these groups tend to be torn apart as they come into money, especially if the projects are big enough to where people can choose camps."

It wasn't always like this; Caridade used to have more respect. The president, Antonio, despite his alcoholism, was considered a brilliant day hospital nurse. Fevereiro and Bakari appeared on Mozambican television, letting journalists into their homes to report on the situations of HIV patients. Carlitos had regular engagements on the local radio station, talking about the importance of testing and the effects of treatment. Luisa attended Ministry of Health meetings as a stand-in for HIV patients and appeared on stage at political rallies, giving speeches about how the government needed to treat patients better. Members often reminisced about the old days. Fevereiro recounted this story about the association before they had NGO funding:

Brada [brother]! Back in those days, Dr. Cesário would come here and pick us up, three, four, or five of us and take us to the [provincial health] training center. This was what he did when the new nurses didn't believe anyone with HIV would actually tell someone else that they had it. We would sit in front of the class, drinking *Coca* [Cola], and answering their questions. How did we get it? What do we do about it? How is it possible that we're even surviving?! I tell you, it really opened their eyes [he gestures as if he is opening his own eyes with his fingers]. This is what we liked to do, be seen and open up people's eyes. (Fevereiro, secretary of Caridade)

Talk of what Caridade used to be was common. "People, residents from this neighborhood, used to bring their children to us," Falume told me, "and we would take them to the hospital because they were scared to go." The subject came up because we had a small visitor who had wandered into the office compound with a couple of his friends. Motioning for the child, who was maybe eight or nine years old, to come closer to where we were seated, he put his arm on the boy's shoulders and continued: "This youngster here almost didn't make it. His very father is a member of this association—HIV positive—but wouldn't take the child for treatment. Now look at him! [The child smiles at Falume and glances sheepishly at me.] Look at his arms! He's healthy. Now, bring me some of these people who say Caridade never did anything for anybody" (Falume, Caridade member).

After more time with the group, I began to understand more about what happens, daily, around Caridade's office. Some activists only showed up on payday. Others, usually unpaid, treated the office like home. Formal meetings rarely happened. The monthly meetings that the association claimed on its progress reports were fabrications. By the time an association-wide meeting was called, I had been in Pemba for three months. A supervisor from RENSIDA in Maputo was coming to collect data on the UNICEF project and expected to attend a group meeting. When it started, most members were there, but neither the president nor the vice-president had shown up yet. Falume, president of the assembly, laid out the agenda. First, they were to talk about Action Aid money and a new project that would be implemented. Second, they were to talk about Christian (me) and the purpose of his research. Third, they needed to discuss the UNICEF project with Gibson, who was here from Maputo—but, like the other leaders, he wasn't yet present at the meeting.

The yard was full of about fifty people, some crowded onto the few benches and chairs, but most of them were standing. I recognized about half of these people who made regular appearances at the office. Many others had met me when I visited for my predissertation research a couple of years back. I was offered a place on a bench because I was going to be speaking. The atmosphere was peaceful as Falume told the group about "Stepping Stones," an Action Aid–sponsored program for members to have meetings with neighborhood associations all over the city. Invitations would be sent to the *presidentes dos bairros* (neighborhood presidents), who would set up locations for the meeting to occur. The topic would be "living positively with HIV/AIDS," and Caridade members would facilitate the discussion. Drinks and snacks would be provided. So far, the members were quiet and there were no questions. Falume asked me to introduce myself, and I gave a brief summary of my research goals—to investigate the importance of HIV treatment and the role of the association in the lives of its members. I discussed my nationality, university, and role as a student and anthropologist. Some people nodded their heads, and others appeared completely disinterested. I sat down and Falume asked if there were any comments.

Hands shot up and murmurings came from the crowd. At first I wondered if the comments would be about me, but they weren't. Simao, one of the association's founding members, stood up and spoke:

> There are some people in this association who think they are better than others. Let me just remind everybody that activists are not members, so they shouldn't get the same things that members get. We don't need this kind of language where people put each other down. What I mean is that some activists have said, "I am the coordinator of such and such a program, and others don't mean anything to this association, and I can take money when I want." Some of us have been here for a long time, and we are being left out when we are supposed to get things. (Simao, founding Caridade member)

The previous evening, Simao had called what he termed a "founder's meeting," that took place at the office, where only original members of the association were invited. It was about some bicycles that were given to Caridade by Action Aid and distributed to certain members without the consent of the entire group. Simao and his friends didn't get bicycles, but others, including the leaders and the activists, did.

A number of people at the current meeting were upset about this perceived unfair transaction, and the noise level rose considerably after Simao's comment. As Falume tried to quiet the crowd, the association's president, Antonio, walked in through the entrance to the compound. He was wearing a white shirt with the phrase "Follow the Leader" in red written in English across the front. Antonio's gait made me suspect what I later confirmed with Carlitos—he had been drinking. He took a seat next to Falume up front, aware of the nature of the protest but not of Simao's exact comments, and began directing the meeting:

> What we need here is honesty and equality and for people to be serious about the work we are doing in my, I mean our, association. I say our association because we all know that associations are composed of many people. Now, normally there is no way to know if people are lying until we catch them. But I am the president here. I know things that others do not, and I have certain rights that others do not. I happen to know that there are some people robbing money [he looks directly at the accountant, Bakari]. When this sort of thing happens, they will be taken out of the association, just the same way as it happened last time. (Antonio, Caridade's president)

At this statement, shouts of anger arose from the group that elevated emotions even higher than before. In part, this was a direct response to the threat of removing people from the association. It was, additionally, an affirmation (and outrage) of what Simao had just acknowledged—that some people think themselves better than others. The president himself had received one of the bicycles in question. Zealous, Bakari the accountant stood up and accused the president of walking directly into his office and taking money out of the association's coffers. He was rebuked by the president and stormed off of the patio into his office.

Another member, Ana Maria, stood up and began denouncing what she claimed to be unfair treatment. Returning from visiting family in Maputo, she learned that her paid activist position had been taken by someone else, and she found herself unemployed. "I told Luisa [the coordinator of the UNICEF school project] that I needed to take this month off, but when I got here, this one [she points to Bryson, seated next to me] was doing my job." Bryson, not HIV positive, and new to the association, was Luisa's younger brother. The implication was that his appointment to her paid activist position was an act of nepotism. As Ana Maria continued to defend herself, Bryson asked to borrow my phone and sent a text message with it. A few minutes later Luisa, who had been absent from the meeting (Bryson told me she was sleeping), stormed into the compound, fingers raised, and shouting. She directly confronted Ana Maria and the two traded remarks in Makua. Others had to break the two women apart, and palpable tension grew throughout the yard.

Because of this confusion, I slinked away from the patio and joined the crowd of youngsters at the back, near the latrines and farthest away from the melee. There were about eight of them, all teenagers, who had joined Caridade as members of a drama group for prevention education. They had just won an award for a skit they carried out at a government function on Mozambican Women's

Day. The prize was a roll of *capulana* cloth, six meters of that colorful and pat-terned African material commonly seen wrapped around the waists and heads of women. It was enough to either make a series of matching outfits for the drama group or sell it in the market for a small sum. However, President Antonio had stolen it from the office—I witnessed this myself. Against the protests of Carlitos and Falume, who tried to stop him, he strapped it to his motorcycle and drove away with it a few days ago. The president frequently helped himself to items in the office if he could sell them to fund his drinking habit—phones that people left in the office to charge, notebooks, power cords, an electric fan. He had, in the recent past, helped himself to project-related items also, a soccer ball and a box of pens destined for schoolchildren in one of the northern districts. Given his behavior, it wasn't difficult for me to believe Bakari's claim that Antonio helped himself to the money in the office as well.

From what I had observed about Luisa's behavior, it wasn't difficult for me to believe that Ana Maria had been unfairly removed from her activist job in favor of Bryson, Luisa's brother. Over the couple of months I had been conducting ethnography with the association, Luisa's absence was more common than her presence, and I was beginning to think of her as corrupt. She was never around the office. Seeing her or speaking to her required going to her home or calling her phone. She showed up in the office only on payday or when important visitors made appointments with her. When letters arrived at the office, she demanded that they be brought to her home for her to read, responding directly in the name of the group and without consulting others. I would occasionally run into Luisa at government meetings or in the offices of the Núcleo or of MONASO, talking with the bosses.

She could also be seen taking taxis around town and sometimes would disap-pear for days. We would later discover that she had been sent for some kind of training in another district or another province, in the name of Caridade, but she never reported back to the group about the results nor passed on informa-tion. The normal process for the group to select who was chosen for these kinds of engagements was always bypassed. In order to continue spending time with Luisa, I visited her frequently in her home, where discussion centered on HIV/AIDS and politics in Mozambique. However, I noticed that she also had begun to drink steadily. One evening, she made advances toward me, but I refused. After that, our relationship never fully recovered. Ana Maria's complaint against her today was a synthesis of what the group wished they could tell Luisa—that her antics were obvious and that she was using the group to install her own friends and family members into paid positions. When the president, Antonio, wasn't treating the association as his own personal bank and private resource, then Luisa, the vice-president, was busy driving the group into a state of oligarchy.

As I meditated upon these problems, waiting in the back of the crowd with the teenagers, I realized that Gibson, the boss from RENSIDA in Maputo, had quietly joined the meeting. It seemed that others began to recognize his presence around that time, and the loud, disrespectful remarks ceased. He didn't speak at first; he just leaned against the wall. I thought he was playing with his phone but later realized he was taking notes. As attention settled on him, he began to address another conflict, one he must have already known about because it wasn't brought up in the meeting.

It involved an accusation from Antonio that Luisa had stolen money from him. Gibson addressed this by grilling Antonio about particular budget numbers, which resulted in the president floundering on all types of information, making him seem untrustworthy about the money in question. The president looked foolish and said nothing in reply. "*Somos iguais* [we are all equal]," said Gibson, speaking again to the whole group, "so what is the fighting really about?" He went on to explain that the association needed better reporting or it risked losing UNICEF funding and appointed three people to collect and compile reports from the school initiative. Later, in a private conversation, Gibson told me that these internal conflicts were not RENSIDA's problem, that they have no control over these issues, and that they are to be worked out on the local level. RENSIDA, even with such interest in the group's data and project success, apparently espoused a "hands-off" approach to the internal conflicts Caridade was experiencing.

Caridade was even more complex than I initially supposed, especially in terms of people agreeing and working together in a unified way. I began to wonder, "Who benefits from this sort of chaos?" This is a question already answered by other scholars and researchers of group behavior. Commenting on the famous Northfield Experiments, a study on group psychology that took place during World War II in England, Miller and Rose (1994) suggest that conflict within the therapeutic community can be productive for someone but rarely for the group itself. The Northfield Experiments were geared toward reintegrating soldiers with psychological casualties back into the military. The first Northfield Experiment, intended to be an indication of what occurs "naturally" and without the imposition of structure, involved what were called "leaderless group tests." These included the intentional absence of appointed leaders, external direction, or authority to allow, ostensibly, the qualities of undiscovered or unrecognized leaders to emerge.

One unique finding was that the most effective leaders were those more in tune with the needs of the group, not those with simply the highest military or educational rank (Kraemer 2010). In addition, observers (or really, interventionists) found that by coaching certain individuals—those with stronger wills or who felt they deserved to lead—they could send them back into the group and repurpose its activities according to their own advantage. The end result was anarchy, infighting, and a more, not less, dysfunctional group than before. Because solidarity was not attained, and group goals warped, the experiment was deemed a failure. This first experiment was aborted after just six weeks. But as Miller and Rose note, a new type of insight was exposed—"the understanding that the group and its dynamics could now be acted upon and used by others both to reveal and to transform the individuals who comprised it" (1994: 41).

In Caridade's case, the group's top leaders were also the apparent top sources of angst and distress for others there. Antonio, a nurse and an employee of the state, and Luisa, a veteran of association and activist trainings in the country, were also both most frequently at the center of group conflict. Their motives were highly questioned by the group, leaving members in an unstable emotional state, and through its leaders, the group appeared most penetrable from the outside. The president and vice-president's positions as program coordinators made them vulnerable to criticism, as they made decisions and statements that came across as nondemocratic and authoritative. The leaders appeared to occupy a rank second to none in a kind of pecking order, and it is this that drew the ire of other members. This feature of the group effectively contradicted the statement of Gibson—undoubtedly an authority figure and flown in from Maputo—that everyone here was equal. His stance, that RENSIDA did not interfere in these situations, positioned Caridade in many ways as its own little Northfield Experiment, complete with the "leaderless group test"—the noninvolvement of the country's national association leaders in this intragroup conflict.

Another important finding from the Northfield Experiments was that the group was not isolated from its surroundings but that therapeutic communities "have a defined direction of activity which is determined by the social system in which they are located" (Miller and Rose 1994: 44). This is another way of stating that the group is under normative pressures but takes the concept further—the group is absorptive of and serves to reflect the culture and social forces that surround or inform it. This has obvious applications for activists in relationship with the state. If the state wants the group to be productive, then that line of thinking will be pursued. If, on the other hand, the state wants an unorganized group—and this actually may have been the case in Mozambique, such that a countercultural activism could not flourish—then the chances the group will be maladjusted are much higher.

Wilfred Bion (1991), directly involved with the designs and chronicling of the Northfield Experiments, told us that the task of those who want to work with the group, in these instances, is to pursue it to the point of disturbing its dynamics and performance. When that happens, the group ceases to evoke therapy. Instead, it evokes "primitive psychotic anxiety" (39). In that sense, the shouting, posturing, and arguing over benefits and bicycles in Caridade are incriminating of both the group itself and those who support it or use it for the data it provides. The group "absorbs," to some extent, the practices of African elites—the government. There are normative pressures for the group to *not* be unified and even for members to cheat or cut corners in their efforts to survive or get ahead.

As I came to work with and know more about Caridade, it became clear that some group members engaged in practices of fraud. Two accountants had pilfered the group's bank accounts and left. Leaders and program coordinators regularly forged receipts for project expenses, pocketing the money. They would claim travel money when travel was never performed. They would punish lower-level activists by withholding salaries and keeping them for themselves. Income generation projects were pillaged. Community gardens were razed overnight, goats stolen from the project pens, and chicken-raising projects staged and money claimed in order for individual members to pay for meager expenses, including household rent and occasional alcohol drinking sessions. Notebooks, pens, and pencils—supplies for members to attend adult education courses—were sold by the box or packet in the local markets. If the group codifies or mirrors what goes on around it, then, like the Mozambican state itself, and even some of its donors (Hanlon 2004), Caridade promoted and lived a lifestyle of corruption.

All this was considered not only relatively normal and socially acceptable but even enviable. Other associations and support groups wanted to be like Caridade. What the group did, its practice of fraud, embodied what, in Mozambican Portuguese, is called *to mafiar*—to defraud others for personal gain. It is a technique, a concept on par with the *pedido* I described in chapter 2. Both the *pedido* and *mafiar* are frequent practices in Mozambican society. They point to insecurity, or what Bion (1991), as noted above, called "primitive psychotic anxieties." Caridade espoused them both and espoused them well.

It is important to understand the term *mafiar* in order to contextualize Caridade's position, and that of other AIDS associations, in this society—this is what AIDS activism passes for and consists of on the ground and in the field. *Mafiar* is a slang Portuguese verb in its infinitive form, derived from what we know in English as "the mafia." It literally means to deceive others via illegal or questionable practices but in a particular manner. It implies a concerted effort on the part of a network of individuals and so differs from the basic concept of being deceived, lied to, or fooled—the term in that case is *enganar*. It differs also from *robar*, the simple act of robbing or being robbed. Let me explain how *mafiar* is different. If I get charged too much from the woman selling tomatoes in the market, this is simple deception. I got fooled—*ela me enganou* (she deceived me). If people break into my house and steal my radio, *eles me robaram* (they robbed me).

If, on the other hand, an enterprising businessman buys up a section of beach property that was previously considered off limits to others, and is able, with the blessing of the government and other local businesses, to acquire the proper permits and materials needed to construct a profitable hotel or restaurant, *ele nos mafiou* (he "mafiared" us). He both deceived us and robbed us, collectively, of something that is not just mine but ours—the ancestral land in and around Pemba City rapidly being taken up for private gain. *Mafiar* combines the arts of deceiving and robbing and applies it to teamwork. Caridade, and AIDS associations like it in and around Pemba City, were considered by some to be mafia-like organizations. This had to do with their involvement in government and NGO-funded projects—the "institutional isomorphism" of the group with other groups, including the state, viewed as predatory or poised to empower personal economies over collective ones.

If there were "normative pressures" at work on Caridade, we do not need to look far to discern their origin. Victor Igreja's description (2008) of Mozambican parliamentary procedures—complete with aggressive posturing, finger pointing, yelling, and walkouts—is not a far cry from the scene I just described during Caridade's meeting. In spite of sharp personal disagreements, leaders of the ruling Frelimo political party maintain their power via access to outside networks of influence and defending the interests of an upper middle class vis-à-vis other social and political groups. It is the unspoken claim of these, as Jason Sumich (2013) describes them, "African elites"—those with the ability to continue developing relationships with lucrative political and foreign actors—that if they lose power, then the alternative (Renamo, or another less-well-connected political party) would be even more corrupt, more disastrous, and less able to negotiate well for the productivity of the country and the lifting up of the masses from poverty.

Pitcher (2008) adds to this by suggesting that the Mozambican elite, despite party rhetoric appealing to equality and power to the people, performs well due to backdoor deals and questionable marriages between government and private sector interests, what she terms "smart partnerships" (2008: 140). This refers to the capacity of the government to *mafiar* in Mozambique, as those in power seek to broker deals and sit on the boards of companies invited in to develop the nation's resources or financial sectors. Like the wider culture around it, Caridade is something of a mafia.

What the Northfield Experiments suggested—that a group is penetrable from the outside, especially through its "leaders," and that a group is absorptive, displaying or reflecting the society in which it is entrenched—may be evident in groups like Caridade and their tendency toward "institutional isomorphism." But what about conflict? If the group is productive for outsiders, as the Northfield Experiments suggested, how does conflict fit into that equation?

Why would any entity or actor want to disturb the group's dynamics or impact its performance in this way? How and why might evoking "primitive psychotic anxieties" be desirable, helpful, or contributory to some other agenda or project?

Thinkers and philosophers on neoliberal governance have the answers here: the group does not exist to serve society, or even the group itself, but rather, it exists to serve the *market*. Criminality, efforts to *mafiar*, and examples of dissent and fission within the group are perfectly acceptable. As long as they are well regulated, conflict and criminality are just smaller markets within other, bigger ones (Lemke 2001). Certainly, a penal code exists to catch those who break the rules, but punishments meted out are geared toward controlling the environment rather than the guilty offenders. The result will be more civil society and not less, more associations and not fewer, because as long as these groups exist to serve the market—from the perspective of neoliberal governance—they are not at all problematic. Their proliferation—well regulated, controlled, filtered, or funneled—is a boon to industry.

Caridade's situation had serious implications for the traditional goals of AIDS activism in the area, revising the evangelistic nature of the enterprise and how civil society transforms the rest of society. When new associations began to form in and around Pemba City, in many ways, they modeled themselves on Caridade, the first group they knew that experienced "success." Caridade's many projects and the group's capacity to gain funding, along with its immature capacity for social solidarity, stifled the reasoning of later groups and their innovation in the realm of organizational modeling. A high-profile, low-functioning group like Caridade may have helped seal the fate of others that were to follow. The president of a group in nearby Mecufi, vying to register with the government and become an official association, told me, "We want to be like Caridade, at all of the [government] meetings, able to ask for things. . . . They have a good *mafia*; we want to be part of this *mafia*." Other new groups, like Bem Vindo, which was awarded the EGPAF home-based care contract, took action plans and project proposals from previously successful Caridade documents, substituting their name for Caridade's when submitting them to donors and funders.

Continuing with DiMaggio and Powell's framework for institutional isomorphism, what occurred was "mimetic isomorphism" (1983: 51), where organizations model themselves on those they perceived to be more successful or legitimate. This was especially likely when the goals of a group or movement, like AIDS activism, are poorly understood, ambiguously defined, or hedged in by uncertainty. The three facets of institutional isomorphism discussed here—coercive isomorphism, normative pressures, and mimetic isomorphism—were encouraged and supported by the state and its partners. This is clear from encounters shared during trainings and meetings that associations were expected to attend. What these next encounters that I describe suggest is that the state did what Wilfred Bion proposed is necessary to effectuate an unorganized group—pursue it to the point of disturbing its dynamics and performance, in this case, by inserting itself only in select ways but also by withdrawing and being absent in others.

STANDARDIZED CIVIL SOCIETY

For government, part of the problem with AIDS associations is that they do not function as well as expected. The state was well aware of the kinds of problems that Caridade and groups like it were having. Manuel, the director of the Núcleo (Pemba's Provincial AIDS Council Office), blamed it on the naiveté of group members. Caridade, he told me one day in his office, "never did understand the meaning of *associativismo*. People form these associations for money, and they never learn how to get along," he said. "But it's not just Caridade, it's all of the associations. Cabo Delgado is very behind with associations and *associativismo*." Curiously, the intervention itself, the injection of *associativismo* into the daily lives of average persons, despite causing friction, remains valid and free from criticism. This brings into focus the "social iatrogenesis" initially described by Ivan Illich (1982)—like a nosocomial infection, the problem itself is transmitted through the medium of therapy, help, or assistance. Labeling Caridade, as opposed to the model forced upon the group, as deviant makes it clear that a monopoly has been established—namely, by the government and its bureaucracy. Bureaucracy does not tolerate complaints. It turns them into either opportunities or misdemeanors. The result is a disqualification of whatever doesn't fit, mediated through processes dubbed value-free and objective.

The experts and specialists enforcing such processes seemed to be imposing a burden but not very strictly. There are half-hearted attempts to transpose poor performance into a better system. More and more partners are introduced to assist the group, but none are directly responsible or charged with making substantive changes. There is both more and less supervision. Excuses can be made for failures, success celebrated, and certain people promoted or rewarded. Mozambicans are familiar with this configuration. Discussing the establishment of democracy and democratic governance in northern Mozambique, Harry West (2008) emphasizes this troubling paradox. In the transition from socialism to democracy, people here were simultaneously more *and* less regulated. Just like the postindependence era, the presence and influence of administrators and bureaucrats are ubiquitous, even expanded.

However, what is new with democracy is the hesitancy on their part to take sides and their refusal to adjudicate for fear that blame will be passed on to party political representatives or others in decision-making power. Mozambicans, West notes (2008), are increasingly expected to "govern themselves." The social space provided by *associativismo* is primed for experimenting with what does or does not work in the community but with nobody to blame for what goes wrong besides the beneficiaries. The intervention, despite at times being the very cause of more chaos, remains whole and intact. Repair efforts are directed toward the group, not the model, not toward the concept of *associativismo* or those who promote it.

A plethora of groups and persons are "in charge" of overseeing AIDS associations in the country—the Núcleo; MONASO; the various foreign NGOs, such as EGPAF and Medicos del Mundo, in Pemba. But adhering to this laissez-faire approach, they provide only frameworks, suggestions, and ideas intended to help or assist AIDS activists with carrying out their duties. They rarely, if ever, become personally involved. Meanwhile, technocrats remain largely irresponsible for the effects of this approach, which typically involves providing trainings or workshops to civil society groups. When convenient, credit can be taken for the impacts of this. When inconvenient, hands can easily be washed and new groups created out the ashes of failed ones. Like the agricultural farming cooperatives of old, civil society associations in Mozambique are given plans and structures to which they are told they must conform in order to be recognized as approved partners of the state.

There are also loose guidelines—laid out in what is called "Ministerial Diploma no. 40/2003 of April 2nd"—which govern civil society in Mozambique. This diploma establishes two principles to be followed. The first is called "the Principle of Complementarity" between the government, donors, and civil society associations. This principle allows citizens to create civil society groups, as long as they "comply" with legislation. The diploma also establishes "the Principle of Collaboration," allowing civil society groups access to existing state resources and the decision-making processes of the national health system. This is what justifies AIDS activists sitting in on the meetings of government health committees, for example. This diploma and the principles laid out in it allow, and even demand, that civil society and government be intertwined with each other. Civil society's access to state resources is dependent on the state's access to civil society. This diploma serves as a blanket proclamation that the government has a role and the final say in designating and approving what it considers to be legitimate or official civil society.

The government, then, has the duty to train civil society on how to be effective. The preferred method for this involves the use of "experts" who work for Frelimo or one of the state-organized NGOs. These experts are flown in to Pemba from Maputo and lodged, usually, in the Pemba Beach luxury hotel for the training period. The standard medium for communicating between these experts and local, sometimes illiterate or uneducated, activists involves laptops, PowerPoint presentations, and screen projectors—all tools to which local associations have little or no access. The format for these trainings involves lectures and small groups. Facilitators ask participants to answer questions—such as "What are the requirements to register as an association with the government?"—and the people respond. They may be asked to define certain terms—such as "ethical," "monitoring and evaluation," or "good governance"—and then congratulated when correct or corrected when wrong.

I will present now some slides from one such training, translated from Portuguese, which dictate to the associations what they must do and how they are to behave in order to receive recognition from the government. These slides are taken from the "Good Civil Society Governance" training hosted by the *Mecanismo de Apoio à Sociedade Civil* (MASC, or the Mechanism for Civil Society Support) at the Frelimo party headquarters in downtown Pemba City.

Figure 3.1 defines the stages through which associations must pass in order to officially register their group. It is presented as rigid; groups are advised not to stray from this path. Here, groups are told that the first step to becoming a civil society group is to hold elections in the context of a general assembly, then pick a name for their group. The name must be unique because it will appear in government records and files. The group must then develop what are called "statutes." These expound a mission statement for the association and list out its goals and objectives. The group may then present these to the government—in the case of AIDS associations, to the NGO known as MONASO—for approval. A contract may then be signed between the association and the public, for which the government is signatory. After this, a constitution may be written, laying out the rules by which the group will function. At this point, the group may become officially registered. Their name will be published nationally in the government bulletin—the *Boletim da República*—the same publication that lays

Levels of Management and Good Governance

1. Institutional Level

Steps guiding the official registration of associations

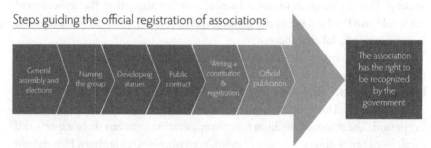

FIGURE 3.1. Formally registering a civil society association

out new laws and directives between from the government to its citizens. At this point, according to the diagram, "the association has the right to be recognized by the government."

This next slide, figure 3.2, harkens back to the organogram presented to Caridade at the beginning of this chapter. Here, the association is educated on the acceptable structure of the group, which includes institutional, organizational, and operational tiers (like a corporation). The group is expected to have three levels, with workers on the bottom, leaders on the top, and another set of managers in the middle. Interestingly, "all" the association's activities belong on the bottom level, but the decisions are to be made on the top. The slide dictates that the group should be hierarchically structured and that its activities should flow not from the needs of the community, necessarily, but from above.

Members have rights and responsibilities, as laid out in figure 3.3. This slide suggests that members must participate in their own activities for the group to succeed. Voting and elections figure prominently in the formulation. It is recommended that the group function like a little version of Frelimo or another political party, with stipulations that members must try hard to agree with one another, make financial contributions, and share their viewpoints. The designers

Relationship between Management Levels and Governance

- **The Institutional/Strategic Level:** The highest level of governance shaped by the constitution, vision, and mission of the association and the rights and responsibilities of its members. This is where decisions are defined and taken.

- **Organizational/Tactical Level:** This level unites the others, drives actions, and settles disputes between them. It reconciles the institutional and operational levels with one another.

- **Operational/Technical Level:** This level is linked to the daily problems of the association. It is the level where all of the association's activities are carried out and is the level responsible for the proper functioning of the association.

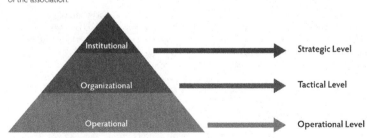

FIGURE 3.2. Levels of an association

of the training, who represent the government, believe that group members must be encouraged to be "active" participants, which counters the notion that the group was formed out of authentic need or solidarity. By default, groups must be "nurtured" to exist and encouraged to take action, not against the government or its laws, but in the world of the group itself, its own meetings and miniature parliament sessions.

In the final slide presented in this three-day training (which I've omitted here, because it's mostly blank), associations are asked to complete an action plan for the changes they identify as required for the group to improve. The "Action Plan for Change" requires the group to identify a problem, followed by stating the ways it can be resolved. They were told to complete the following columns: "questions to address," "the action to begin taking," "names of the responsible persons," "the time frame for execution," and "the necessary resources." During this session of the training, members were divided into groups according to their associations. In my group, Caridade members quickly zeroed in on the "necessary resources" column and identified the need to purchase their own office so that rent would no longer have to be paid to the government agency who owned the current space. For this, only money was needed, and no plans were put forward on how to obtain it.

When the groups came together again to present our action plans to the room, not a single plan, including ours, failed to list money as a necessary resource. Other groups identified additional material items as their "question to address." A car, a computer, and a new latrine were among the desired prizes. The training, apparently, did not help the associations to innovate, nor did they

Rights and Responsibilities of Assocations

- **Member responsibilities and participation**—the members of the association must actively participate in the association's activities to help it reach its objectives.

Rights	Responsibilities
· To vote and to be elected.	· Contribute to the association's success.
· To participate in all of the association's activities.	· Participate in meetings and elections.
· Access to all files, books, and documents.	· Comply with decisions made by the majority of members.
· Call together a meeting or assembly when necessary.	· Vote in elections.
· Ask for clarification from the administrative council and/or the executive director.	· Adhere to pledges made to the association.
· Share and give opinions and ideas.	· Remain informed about the activities of the association.
	· Denounce failures when they occur.
	· Pay dues and fees to the association.

FIGURE 3.3. Rights and responsibilities of associations

feel encouraged to do so. They already knew money was one of the best solutions, a fact nobody doubted even prior to the start of the week-long affair. The training stopped there, deploying abstract ideas but without generating suggestions for pursuing loans, grants, or business opportunities. The trainers packed up their computers and projectors and flew back to Maputo the next day. Having received their own per diems and salaries but changing nothing for the civil society groups in Pemba City, they were able to include Caridade and other associations on their final reports as successfully "trained."

In *The Anti-politics Machine*, James Ferguson (1994: 259) notes that "development" of the nation comes as a package of standard available inputs, entailing lack of diversity, locked into unimaginative or misleading action plans. The reasons address management concerns more than social or economic progress. Any deviation from a preapproved standard becomes more difficult for a routinized bureaucracy to implement and evaluate. The training of civil society in Mozambique, just like many other "projects" in this context, encourages institutional isomorphism. Any version of civil society unlike that put forth in these kinds of trainings is less likely to be recognized by the government, less likely to get funded, less likely to have needs met or be seen as a legitimate "partner." While Ferguson reminds us that the precedence for applying formulas and proscriptions to international development projects in southern Africa is well entrenched, what may be unique in Mozambique is the extent to which the state goes to treat civil society as part of the bureaucracy rather than an alternative to it, or as an extension of governance rather than a compass for it.

What the state intends by this maneuvering is impossible to discern from my data alone; however, the effects of it are clear. Given what has occurred between governments and AIDS activists in other countries—like TAC in South Africa—it was no coincidence that the Mozambican state sought to position itself as overseer (a mini-God, or "demiurge"). The potential for civil society to rebel or complain was met not with open antagonism but with claiming to be a reliable source of assistance or help. To temper any "threat" against itself, the Mozambican state simply upheld a long-standing tradition of close involvement with special interest groups, just like the old agricultural farming cooperatives and the *grupos dynamizadores*. Articulated as *associativismo*, the result was certainly "antipolitical." By doing this, the state appealed to the same values espoused by politically active AIDS activists—seeking inclusion rather than exclusion and demanding the right to lobby and approach the state with their concerns—but in a way that was preordained to be manageable and tolerable for bureaucrats and elites.

The effect was regulation, the containment of AIDS activism within a box of apparent equity that did not, on the surface, seem unreasonable. However, the requirements given by the state for the official recognition of AIDS (and other) associations acted as a kind of glue to bring together and harden the trinity of institutional isomorphisms—coercion, normative pressure, and mimeticism. Stressing this uniformity stifled and choked off diversity, discouraging innovative or entrepreneurial alternatives to the accepted standard, and impacting competing visions for the future. The next training that I will describe highlights the nonresponse of the facilitator to the felt needs of the group, sharing, reemphasizing, and reinforcing a conclusion drawn from the last encounter—that associations are probably better off without the trainings and government "experts" than with them.

Enormous resources, most likely from donor money, were invested in these kinds of trainings for which the state takes credit, positioning itself as patron and benefactor. Through this kind of "neopatrimonialism" (Pitcher, Moran, and Johnston 2009) the government tries to solicit consent and obedience, expecting compliance and acquiescence from structural subordinates but without the real right to demand it or the resources to back it up. Next, I draw additional attention to how inelegant this proves to be on the ground and in actual practice. The "little" protests in the following scenario are the seeds of the larger one that I will describe in chapter 5.

"LITTLE" PROTESTS AND THE WORKSHOPOCRACY

"Conflict can lead to war, so we must avoid conflict in our associations," said the government-hired trainer who nobody knew and who had flown in from Maputo for the day. I wondered if he used these words on purpose, given Mozambique's twenty-year-long armed struggles, to evoke images arousing nationalist emotions. He represented the Frelimo party and had arrived just a couple of months before the next presidential election. The title of this training was "Effective Association Building, Management, and Leadership." "And what is the cause of conflict?" he asked.

Abacar, an older man, shouted back, "Gender inequality! Women have too much power in the home."

Another person remarked, "Troublemakers! Too many people want to help themselves and not others!"

Yussuf, an outspoken guy said, "The president!" Positive group consensus developed around this last suggestion, and a symphony of heads nodded yes.

In the back, another man shouted out, "*Uhemia hemia!*" (in Makua, "authoritarianism"). He continued, "The president forgets he is a member of the association and thinks he is above everyone else." Grunts of agreement and approval echoed through the room. The trainer nodded and said thank you, then clicked a button on his computer forwarding to the next slide in his PowerPoint presentation. Neither the word "president" nor "authority" was on it. "Transparency is the problem," he said, as if no comments had ever been made.

I thought of how the World Bank defines transparency and accountability as essential to good economic reform (World Bank 1992). Perhaps some of the Bank's ethics—demanding disproportionate accountability from below rather than from above—had arrived at this level of society, implanted in the trainer's mind.

The trainer continued, "We must show the available resources and how they are used. Look at Mama Fátima here. When I saw her exit the taxi this morning, as an association member, I could have thought she was using our resources for her own benefit and that she was stealing when actually she is not. Assuming she used the association's money is bad accountability. Good accountability reduces conflict and bad thinking." He went on to talk about the importance of submitting receipts to justify daily expenses. This tendency was common in the trainings I witnessed in Pemba. After soliciting the group's opinion on a topic, the trainer barely addressed it and moved on to another issue.

In this case, the group moved on as well. There were other concerns to bring up. "When we submit documents to the government, it always takes them so long to respond," mentioned a woman wearing a hijab (Marilia).

The trainer smiled. "That's because you don't understand. You have no comprehension of sectoral interdependence. They will tell you to expect the issue to be resolved in 45 days, but it will often take longer because there are a lot of people who have to approve your request, make sure it is safe, not threatening to others."

Dinho, who was in a community lawyer's association, stood up. "We have been waiting for one and a half years to hear back about running a minibus transport business out of our association!"

Building the excitement, another man stood and said, "Our association has been waiting two years for permission to put a sign up in front of our office to be officially recognized by the government!"

Alberta, a former Caridade member, loudly added, "When we need the ambulance from the hospital to pick up a sick patient, we find it is stopped at a bar."

"So there is conflict here?" asks the trainer.

"Yes!" came a unison response from the group.

For a brief moment the trainer looked out the window. He exhaled heavily, and I believe I saw a quick look of exhaustion sweep across his face. He then turned back around and advanced his PowerPoint slide, never responding to any of the concerns just mentioned. Instead, he continued defining terms. "A leader," he said, "is someone who influences others, while a manager is an implementer."

Seemingly undeterred, someone brought the topic back to conflict. "It is these very people—leaders and managers—who want money without doing any work."

"Ah, but this is interpersonal conflict," said the trainer. "We think it is not group conflict, but it is. We think it is not a problem."

The emotional distance between the trainer and the group grew as he ignored their comments, and the "we" statements made the exchange seem like he was talking to children. He stuck to his slides and definitions and entered into a rehearsed speech about Samora Machel and Eduardo Mondlane. According to the trainer, these founders of Frelimo and heroes of Mozambican independence knew that "when confronting your enemy, you must have a plan, a strategy." He picked up an orange. "One association member wants to make a cake with this orange, the other wants to make fruit. What do we do? Do we split it in half, or do we do something with the orange that the other member doesn't want to do?"

Perplexed by this nonsensical example, participants at the training remained stoic. No answers came forth. "This is the kind of thing we must think about," continued the trainer. "Do we confront this problem right now, as it is? Or do we delay and postpone the debate?" Time began to move slowly as vocal participation on the part of the group dwindled. It started to seem like the trainer was trying to train himself. Grasping at straws, he asked, "Why should the president have to ask someone to clean, when that person should already know her role? She should clean without being asked! We must reinforce our roles in our associations." As the day was winding down, he again touched on a sensitive topic. "What about membership fees and monthly dues, can we kick someone out of the association for not paying these?"

"Yes," says the group, unenthusiastically. By now, there was little effort to call attention to the white elephant that the trainer just let into the room— associations were unable to either make ends meet with monthly dues or enforce their payment. Even before the training was over, people began to filter out of the room. Some didn't even return for the free Coca-Cola and snacks at the end of the day.

Commenting on the rise of civil society in Tanzania, Kelsall suggested that the governmental began to institute a "workshopocracy" (2002: 604)—the use of forums like trainings and workshops to address the needs of grassroots groups but in ways removed from authentic public interests. This worked well for the government, which used them to demonstrate its apparent support of civil society initiatives. Every training or workshop carried out justifies the state in the eyes of donors. Regardless of how hollowed out the subject material may be or how vacant the substance of discussion and debate, what is important is that the training be done, implemented and noted on official forms, spreadsheets, or reports. Trainings and workshops become window dressing for what Kelsall calls "politics of the veranda" (598). Figuratively speaking, funders, managers, and administrators walk by, catching glimpses of civil society involvement, and see politics being aired in public, even though on the inside of the building the room is empty and devoid of any real political change. This is one way to think about "bad" workshops.

Another way to think about workshops is as an imposition on the concept of "self." Discussing the use of workshops with AIDS activists in West Africa, Nguyen (2010) points out how they resonate with neoliberalism because they "steer" activists in particular directions—toward processing their feelings, engaging with self-help literature, motivating participants to approach life in a more positive light, and debriefing with others to remold their perceptions of bad experiences. The implication of some who have studied the dynamics of testimonials and confessional technologies among HIV-positive persons (Robins 2004; Robins 2006) is that initiatives geared toward skills building or crisis alleviation are an overstepping of boundaries, subtle means of thought control, and limiting in scope.

From this perspective, any outside effort to "transform" the "subjectivity" of patients comes across as not good enough, too uniform in its application, and less effective than enabling group participants to become politically involved and engage the governance structure as well-educated activists. What I would like to suggest, however, is a slightly different approach—the trainings and workshops that cause the most damage dash people's hopes by mocking their choice to become involved with civil society in the first place. The most distressing manifestation of a "neoliberal workshopocracy" is devoid of any useful techniques at all.

Besides emboldening the state to treat all civil society unimaginatively and uniformly, what the "workshopocracy" really brings into focus—what truly needs to be addressed—is any element of nondemocracy at work. This has less to do with whatever icebreakers, group discussion techniques, or lay psychotherapy exercises are being used than it does with treating participants like children or worthless, passive consumers. What the poorly implemented workshop demonstrates to civil society groups is how limited their options are and how little effort the state has to put forth in order to dismiss them. This is a function of poor quality, bad design, and the reckless selection of facilitators or implementers. It carries with it an enormous weight—of fatalism, discouragement, and frustration—for activists who are now led to believe that, in terms of "partnering" with their government, this is as good as it gets.

Association members in Pemba City would have been much better off *with* workshops that successfully diffused proven self-help techniques than with ones feigning government interest and guidance. It is, in a word, demoralizing to make workshop participants feel as if all current and future efforts of their association or group might ultimately come to naught. Trainings or workshops that deepen the reach of the state by infusing self-governance techniques or superficial notions of self-esteem deserve scrutiny in their capacity to require participation in exchange for benefits. However, the most disempowering trainings of all exclude even those who attempt to be included, robbing even those who choose to participate of their benefits, making even their self-determination—often times this is the most people can offer—into just another tool for deradicalization and instrumentalization.

CIVIL SOCIETY EXISTENTIALISM

Caridade's formation, not as a support group but as a state-recognized AIDS association, has been more harmful to the group than it has been helpful. Rendered more visible to the state through its voluntary participation—its adoption and allegiance to particular projects and activities and its agreement to be a partner (in principle) but subordinate (in reality) to other, more powerful actors—makes it a target among other targets similar in function and status who acquiesce to this type of oversight and management. The impotence of the group appears in some ways balanced by its prior and continuing potential, its rise from the recesses of the *bairro* and the clinic, its composition primarily of authentically uneducated and promisingly compassionate activists, members, and volunteers. Its original orientation as community-centered and patient-powered characterizes the group as a very real and tangible version of civil society—at its best, a true success story. The challenge is not how to move beyond this but whether it can be regained.

When civil society becomes a victim of central government planning, the apparent dichotomy of traditionally imposed categories of analysis—the tension between the government and the individual (or in this case, the individual "group")—are not really of principle concern nor the ultimate malefactor. The disaster here is not outside influence, it is the incapacity for all involved to follow a singular rule of law. The group's freedoms and its "rights" and "responsibilities" are presented as limitations, but the government (and its partners), in contrast, gives itself free reign, positioning itself as answerable to none, a minor God, a demiurge. It is in the abstract concept of civil society that this is most damaging. The group is treated as existential, set in motion but with undetectable, invisible, imposed boundaries—given "help" that is meticulously interested but also coldly detached. The group, in actuality, need not consent, agree, or obey, unless it really wants something in return—a contract or a deal.

Fascination with "technologies of the self" as a brutal imposition is misplaced here because it is not the primary mechanism of control. People do not "give in" all that easily to targeted attempts at channeling their behavior, attitude, or lifestyle. Instead, this is achieved by the state (or its partners) in the self-appointed role of overseer, regulatory commissioner, and provider of favors. Ironically, more, not less, discipline is needed on the part of some actors. Those who *mafiar*, conduct bad trainings, and control the group via external and elite alliances devoid of merit but not influence actually *do* need to "govern themselves" better. Doing so would allot them more, not less, freedom. The subtle process of integration, of civil society becoming more like government, of individuals becoming leaders or getting trained is not to be resisted if it leads to better overall accountability. If it doesn't, however, then it must be altogether rejected. If anyone can break the rules, then everyone must start again, until some system or another actually works. We may be in a phase where this is warranted. It is really the only way out of a "neoliberal" confluence, when the group finds itself hopelessly answerable and subservient to others.

This, then, is civil society existentialism: groups such as AIDS associations represent, presumably and in the abstract, automatic freedom from despotism and tyranny, yet their laissez-faire existence is mythical and impossible to attain. The group cannot be wound up, like a clock or a watch, and left on a table alone to do its work. Someone or something will always stop by to try to tinker with it. The group, then, may be better off in a protectionist or isolationist mode, set apart from development projects, action plans, experts, and funding. Otherwise, from the point of view of the state or other regulator, it not only needs but also deserves some form of external guidance and will never truly function on its own. Since that is the case, when a third party inevitably comes into play, it is often able to flout all the rules. Skirting along the periphery of regulation, trainers, association presidents, African elites, paid consultants, and others who come across as "in charge" are equally capable of both subterfuge and empowerment. The choice is largely theirs and not the group's.

This third party continues to not only present but also justify itself as some form of interference, making the power of the state visible but in various other questionable ways and venues. Civil society's supposed natural occurrence does not escape the place and time in which it is embedded. The battleground, in such cases, is the concept of "partnership." Therefore, for groups caught up in the throes of civil society existentialism, the way out is to ignore the ruling powers and carry on alone—in a word, to disengage. When both participation and non-participation yield the same results, the answer is a return to an original state, the same one that drew attention to the group to begin with and supplied it with its initial credentials as a grassroots effort, a worthy ally, and a visible target.

The process may be painful because it involves culling and sacrifice—of apparent progress, of projects and salaries, of faux coalitions and haphazard training regimens—in order to return to a stable state, even if appears to be a step backward. The answer for Caridade, and other Mozambican AIDS associations, is simple but unlikely to be sought. It is to make demands on one another rather than outsiders and to consult and negotiate mostly within the group itself, staying true to original goals and objectives.

The impetus for such a strategy is evident in the nature of works undone or as yet unaccomplished. While chasing funding and approval from bodies and entities higher up on the economic food chain, momentum subtly shifts away from the reasons the group was crafted or called into existence to begin with toward ever more bureaucratic tasks and purposes that chip away at the group's meaning and pragmatic function. Having achieved some success and obtained some recognition, the right kinds of thirsts are slaked, particularly those of leaders and decision-makers. Data are exchanged but reported up a ladder of reverse accountability, such that field-level realities get obfuscated or even ignored. Projects that work well in one context are presumed to work equally well in another, such that oversight or needs for adjustment become less of a priority. Efforts break down, never get repaired, and progress falters. The group, if it so chooses, rests comfortably on its laurels while society around it continues to crumble. Challenges persist that under better circumstances could have worked themselves out.

To evaluate AIDS activism and civil society groups we need not look to government bookkeeping, the amount of money allocated to civil society coffers, levels of publicity and public relations success, or how far and wide the name of some community-based organization or NGO has spread. We need only examine the communities themselves, where such groups are situated and active. In the following chapter, I further focus attention on the local situation, the world and culture in which Caridade is embedded, the microcosm where AIDS activism is presumed to be hard at work. The litmus test for civil society—and those who claim to fund and support it—is read and assessed at the heart of the people, towns, and villages of Cabo Delgado Province.

4 · CHALLENGES TO HIV/AIDS ACTIVISM IN THE "SUBUNIVERSE" OF CABO DELGADO

"This rain is for the mango trees, to make their flowers bloom," said Susanna, as the drops began to pelt the tin roof of the association's abandoned chicken coop where we were conducting our interview. The chickens were all gone. That project hadn't worked out well for the association. We sat there together, caged in, getting to know one another as the rain grew heavier. When Susanna was diagnosed as HIV positive, it was because her constant uterine pains had caused her to seek help at the hospital. She described what sounded to me like pelvic inflammatory disease, which can accompany HIV. For six years, her period never seemed to stop, but she didn't really know what was wrong. "I thought that maybe I didn't have any blood left!" she said. The pain led to her sexual abstinence, and as she got skinnier, her first husband left her in her late teens.

Now, because of the pelvic disease, she had entered menopause at the early age of twenty-five. "When you tell people about the virus, it is strange; they think you are nothing." She adjusts the bracelets on her arm with her other hand, maybe nine or ten of them. They are made from parts of unused female condoms, fashioned by removing the synthetic material that normally cups the cervix upon insertion, leaving rings that are almost indistinguishable from some of the cheap imported jewelry found in local markets. Most people here don't like to use condoms, especially the female ones. They often end up as bracelets and as material for making toys (like soccer balls).

Susanna was now in what people call a "traditional" marriage. Having lived with the same man for a few years, the community viewed them as husband and wife. She told me that this new husband "doesn't want to accept that I am positive, I'm certain of this, even when he sees the medicine. I asked him to do a test, and it was negative. Still, sometimes I divorce him, but we always come together again." Susanna refers to a common practice in the area of informally and temporarily separating from a lover as a result of some frustrating aspect of the relationship. About her AIDS association and her medication, she had this to say:

> When I take the medicine, it is very strong. It helps a lot. But sometimes, I can forget, for two or three days, then I really feel terrible. If you can eat well, then the medications are no problem. Otherwise, you feel drunk [she rotates her head, mimicking dizziness]. The association helps, certainly. We can talk together. We are all sick, so nobody is scared. Mama Fátima mobilized us, saying that if we join, the government will help us. We only got food one time, but they gave us *katanas* [machetes] for working in the garden and some mosquito nets. The most difficult thing for me is the poverty. If we had money, we could buy nutritious foods. In the city it is different. There they are fat! (Susanna, AIDS association member)

Her history of long-suffering, concerns about relationships, stigma, and daily survival are common themes for people with HIV in this region, and in a village as small as Mieze (about twenty kilometers from Pemba), "everyone knows you are ill." She continued, "But that doesn't seem to matter to most of these young girls. They say there is no virus and go with many men. As for me, I have no farm. I am just waiting for God to call me . . . *pronto* [I am ready.]."

Carrying on with her old life as best she can, activists like Susanna are the most common "type" of activist in Cabo Delgado Province. She is not making a career or enterprise out of her diagnosis, as some are. But concerned about those "young girls," her statements, and her status as an association member, she indicates more interest than many take in their own condition, as well as that of others. She is concerned about HIV in her community and the status of those who are affected—her AIDS association and similar groups. She verbalizes her wishes that the situation was different, expresses hope and fears over her future, and identifies specific problems that need to be addressed—namely, poverty and access to other resources that are valued but also scarce both for her and for most other Mozambicans.

Not particularly well educated or politically savvy, Susanna is not locally famous or even among the leaders of local AIDS associations. No newspaper articles have been written about her. Neither she nor her group was the subject of books on treatment activism (until now). She is, however, in many respects, representative and symbolic—an "everywoman." There are more Susannas in the world than there are Zackie Achmats (the outspoken TAC founder) or

Magic Johnsons (the retired basketball star). For her, and others like her, to not be included or considered a part of the world of activism is more than just an oversight; it would be an indication that the ranks of so-called AIDS activists are much thinner than we might suppose or are led to believe.

Susanna does not occupy the same world as the stereotypical, cosmopolitan, urban-based activist. She passively waits for help and is more of a consumer than a producer. She has medication, and now she wants other *things* from her government—food and tools. She does not broadcast her AIDS status. She may even be putting her husband at risk, who is either in denial or unaware of his chances of becoming infected. But this does not devalue her contributions or potential to enact change or social justice. Instead, it indicates a hidden world, one unsensationalized and not held up to the public as exemplary, maybe because it doesn't support the preferred narrative in exactly the right way. Susanna, and many other activists in Cabo Delgado—especially those who do not travel or attend workshops and conferences—occupy a "subuniverse" (Berger and Luckmann 1967: 84) of the more popular, politically motivated AIDS world of activism. That world is the one most often written about, with which most of us are more familiar. In this chapter, I will show that socialization in that world has never been completely successful, and many people I encountered in Mozambique, just like Susanna, do not "inhabit" it as certainly as others.

AIDS activism is not a singular, objective, or independent reality but depends, rather, upon point of view and interpretation. It is a social construct, experienced differently by individuals according to their background and everyday life. The political aspect of activism is, much like other "subjectivities," a social construct and intellectual territory that is not, as some might like to believe, either inevitable or accessible. Susanna may never—as Ida Susser (2009) predicts—transition from being a mere "adaptive" activist into a "transformative" one due to some latent ability to organize others or think like an organic intellectual. But that does not make her "less than" other, better-connected AIDS activists.

Her story matters. Cabo Delgado Province matters, not because it is front and center of the AIDS activist movement but for opposite reasons—as a more neutral territory, where people are not as exposed to predeterminations about what is and is not the acceptable role of an activist. Less touched by the world, more isolated and nondescript, Cabo Delgado is a laboratory for testing the limits and claims of treatment activism and for evaluating its reach. Treatment alone—more clinical facilities, better "access" to medication, even the government's signature on more laws and human rights agreements—won't save the people of Cabo Delgado. Change must continue to occur locally. For this, no clear-cut trails have been blazed. Relatively unstructured, support groups flounder for direction, opportunity, and meaning.

Subuniverses of activism are segmented and segregated, highly contextualized, and structured by a variety of criteria: education and the circulation of knowledge; values that may be spiritual or traditional; aspirations for money, resources, or prestige; and aesthetic tastes for food and drink, for social relations and (dis)unity, and even different kinds or types of healing. This chapter is devoted to the subuniverse of AIDS activism in Cabo Delgado Province, particularly through an explication of the challenges HIV-positive persons and activists face in regard to their condition and what they can and cannot do about it. Reality in this context is ladled with contradiction, misunderstandings, and subjective viewpoints about HIV/AIDS and even activists themselves that threaten to disarm the apparent gains of a dominant mode of activism that has emphasized, perhaps to its detriment, the virtues of treatment alone. These are the views of *"ordinary people,"*[1] taken for granted, dismissed, or ignored by the wider world because of their perceived inaccuracies.

Occupying a world that is real to them, for *ordinary people*, Western abstract notions of illness and social solidarity are often little more than reifications, even presumptuous impositions. Biomedical facts and clinical evidence have little sway over their thoughts and actions. They require an activism that is more practical than it is radical. The challenges faced by AIDS activism that I will discuss here are situated in the beliefs of *ordinary people*. They include the following: lingering confusion about the virus, ineffective home-based care programs, antiretroviral treatment abandonment, and the heavy use of alcohol. None of these are easily solvable simply in the context of the clinic, but they might be mitigated in the context of a high-functioning support group—a model for which we still, after all the political hype and international interest, have no clear blueprint or standard. AIDS activism is relevant here, present and at work in its own way, and continues to be sorely needed, not for establishing ephemeral or imagined connections between persons living far apart but especially for the promotion of resilience and inner strength for the *ordinary people*.

LINGERING CONFUSION ABOUT HIV/AIDS AND ACTIVISM

"AIDS is many things that never stop," said one villager with whom I spoke. "It is just another one of those *doencas incognitas* [unknown diseases]." According to Martinez (1989), for the tribes[2] of northern Mozambique—the Makua, the Mwani, and the Makonde—*doencas incognitas* are considered to be the worst types. They are more deadly even than "very serious illnesses" because they are "imported from whites" (154). Disease is often considered to be disgraceful, the result of existential aggression (on the part of God, ancestors, or jealous persons—witches) or a life out of balance: "AIDS comes from God, whatever thing you find comes from God. God gives us everything, including disease and death. The government didn't bring AIDS here, and the government is good. It gives us pills and food. But God and the government are like this [he crosses his fingers and holds them up, indicating togetherness]. It helps God to provide for us. AIDS came here from a white man, a doctor here in the hospital"[3] (Fernando, AIDS association member).

For many Africans, including AIDS activists, disease is often more of a social than a clinical experience, a mystical rather than biological occurrence. HIV—because of the myriad symptoms it presents—is likely to be misdiagnosed or treated in nonclinical settings. What the patient's family is likely to suspect is that a ritual prohibition on food, hygiene, or sex has been violated. What the patient might be experiencing—impaired movement, neuropathy,[4] vertigo, rheumatism, or *ekhumelo ya emphome* (bad blood, as suggested by Susanna, above)—can be resolved by bathing in roots and herbs gathered from the bush, by drinking a similar concoction, or being "vaccinated" with razor blades by a traditional healer. "When I got sick, my son took me to seven *curandeiros* [traditional healers]. They gave me roots, I took a bath, and it helped a little bit. Those who don't believe the government and don't like the hospital say that HIV is just witchcraft. [I ask her if that is what she thinks.] No, but I used to, and many people still do. They don't listen to us when we tell them what we know" (Anifa, AIDS association member).

Also, HIV and AIDS are not local terms. The virus is commonly referred to as *kidudu,* a Makua word designating worms or gastrointestinal stress and an illness caused, purportedly, by bugs or insects in the body. *Kidudu grande* (big kidudu)—an even worse version of the original—is said to be imported from whites. HIV in northern Mozambique fits into the common plague metaphor described by Sontag (1989: 89)—visited upon a society by outsiders, HIV "is understood in a premodern way."

Activists who I interviewed often first heard about HIV from government outlets, like newspaper articles, radio programs, and educational brochures or pamphlets. These sources mention routes of transmission besides just sex, but by drawing equal attention to them, many patients are encouraged to deny that sex was ever a factor in their own infection. One man told me that he got ill after stepping on a dirty syringe and his foot started itching. Another blamed a blood transfusion in the hospital. Another man believed he got infected as the result of a bloody workplace accident and that HIV had entered by air through his open wounds. Several people told me that they got HIV from the unsanitary treatment of a traditional healer. Less than half of those interviewed mentioned sex.

One woman believed that her baby may have given her HIV: "I could have been infected through the umbilical cord of the baby. We were both infected in the same day [her and the baby]. There is no control in the hospital with blood safety. That day the beds were full, so I could have been stuck with used needles"

(Joaquina, AIDS association member). Other association members suggested that cholera, malaria, and tuberculosis were possible ways to acquire HIV. Efforts to educate people, even "activists," about the virus have been insufficient. An enormous gap exists between knowledge that is passed on—by clinicians and educators and in literature and media—that if it hasn't been addressed by now, it may simply never be, at least not in the same old ways.

Some activists in Cabo Delgado intellectualize the virus as a conspiracy theory, a government project designed and generated to bring in money and kill off unwanted populations:

We hear on the radio that *such and such* number of dollars has come to the government to help people with HIV. Where is this money? Why don't we get it? Because it stops in Maputo! Some say that the whites brought [HIV] here. Why don't they have it? Because they brought it for us! The government talks about it, but they [the ministers of parliament] don't have it. That is because they knew about it before, when it was a secret. The last time they came here [to Macomia], they said HIV would be finished by 2010. They can say that because they can control it. (focus group, Macomia hospital)

This disease is new. It doesn't come from here. Nothing the government does seems to help. For them, it is producing money. In this district, we hear that people in that district are getting money. In that district, they hear that we are getting money. We are always told that it is coming, but it doesn't, and they expect us to stay blind about this? What is happening is this virus is balancing out the country; it lets the government kill people they don't want. What they tell these other countries, there [gesturing far away with her hand] is they are helping us. Does it look like I'm being helped to you? (Celestina, AIDS association member)

In Moçimboa da Praia, some passersby of the local AIDS association *Desafio Jovem* (Youth Challenge) believed Americans had brought HIV to Mozambique because the sign outside of the office, which the association was required by its funder to display, read "*AID* from the American People" (which was misconstrued as *AIDS*). In Cabo Delgado, as an international development concern, the virus is very much associated with money and influence. The theories people propagate indicate their unique grasp on the global AIDS industry. This is not up for much debate or argument, and people are not easily swayed on these points.

Activists are considered to be a part of this government project. Enlisted to "work" in their AIDS associations, members of the community do not trust activists and believe they joined their association out of self-interest. "Some of my neighbors say that we [association members] write our names down and the government brings us money. I look healthy, so they don't even think the virus exists or is a problem. When I encourage them to get a test and visit the hospital, they tell me that this is my *negocio* [business], that I get paid when they join the project" (Juma, AIDS association leader). Some do become activists out of self-interest, so when projects die down, so does the association: "This association used to be for projects. That is why I joined. They told us if we did this, then we would get money from raising chickens. But what we also know is that the government must give us medications. They won't let people with HIV suffer anymore. We had a garden, and we had goats, but now we don't and nobody comes anymore to the meetings. Now nobody works. They just come sometimes, sit around like this, and then go home" (Mohamed, AIDS association member). There is also competition between associations and jealousy, especially based on expectations that the government owes something to the association: "In Mieze, we are always told to do 'sustainable projects, sustainable projects.' Well, I never see Caridade doing sustainable projects! In our village, everything falls into the category of *machamba* [garden]. The associations in the city have more opportunities, even though they do lousy work. They all get paid, and we can't even get a tractor" (Aida, AIDS association member).

Activism becomes an element of the activist's livelihood, a way to get money and survive regularly. They feel dependent on the government and NGOs such as MONASO:

> Here we only have land for the garden but nothing else to make it, no seeds, no hoes. We created this group because MONASO told us to. When we got the land, people said, "This garden is for people with HIV." But we still don't have a constitution or statutes, and MONASO won't give us anything else until we do. We want to be like Caridade, at all of the meetings, able to ask for things. [I tell her that Caridade members are also upset with funding and assistance.] Yes, I know, but they have a good *mafia*, we want to be part of this *mafia*. (Rainha, AIDS association president)

Rainha's statement points to the fact that some AIDS associations compete with each other, leading them to focus more on short-term rather than long-term survival.

Stigma against HIV-positive persons—what Mozambicans call *vergonha* (lit. shame)—remains a significant obstacle in Cabo Delgado. When one's HIV positive status is well known, "people won't buy things from you when you are selling in the market. This has destroyed our association because when we make charcoal or cement blocks [for housing and building construction] people pass us by. They go to the others around us and buy what they need. They do not want to support our association. They call us *infectados* [infected]. Everyone there talks bad about us" (Nelson, AIDS association member and organizer of business activities for the group).

Stigma also keeps many people in the area from getting tested. According to one activist, they are "scared of being contaminated, but they don't want to do a test. When you suggest it, they insult you." When asked to elaborate on why *vergonha* is problematic for HIV positives, that concept was frequently linked to the Portuguese word *desprezar* (lit. to despise). Abiba, who lived in a small village, told me, "I stopped taking my medication because I stopped going to the hospital. I stopped going to the hospital because my neighbor *me desprezou* [despised me]. She talked bad about me and told everyone she met about my [HIV-positive] condition. I was ashamed to show my face or even step outside at daytime. This went on for months" (Abiba, ART patient).

While stigma—the proliferation of spoiled identities (Goffman 1986)—is a common experience for many people with HIV, more distressing even than its presence is, perhaps, the incapacity here to construct a counternarrative. The implication that while stigma happens nothing can be done about it is an indication that the achievements of Mozambican AIDS activists are very likely less than ideal and have largely missed the mark. The "newness" of AIDS associations and AIDS activism in Cabo Delgado has been unable to address this and may be quite limited.

The misinformation that circulates about HIV and AIDS—where the disease comes from, the nature of the government's involvement, and confused ideas about who activists are and what they do—certainly makes it seem as if activist efforts to change the society around them have largely failed. It also identifies ongoing current needs, serving as a map and compass for where activism could or should head in the future. There needs to be a reorientation, first among activists themselves. Their empowerment does not lie in seeking the same kinds of resources as the society around them but in addressing crisis recovery in their own lives, to serve not just as examples of good patients but as good residents and citizens overall. They need skills to avoid disease relapse and to manage their situations better. They need not opportunities for obtaining "new" jobs, or philosophies for developing "new" selves, but the chance to regain what was lost and possibilities for normalization (Philbin 2014).

For attitudes and knowledge in society to shift, for *ordinary people* to embrace accurate structures of plausibility concerning HIV, AIDS associations must be stronger and more effective but not necessarily more politically active or geared toward money. They must be able to convince one another of objective truth without falling prey to substandard "knowledge." These changes are not likely to come from NGOs or the government but from activists themselves. If they are unable to generate relationships and resilience rather than simply income, and dignity rather than competition, they may remain sidelined and grow increasingly irrelevant, even becoming—in and of themselves—obstacles to patient rights and progress.

INEFFECTIVE HOME-BASED CARE PROGRAMS

"We want to extend home-based care to another ten districts this year," said Manuel, the coordinator of Pemba's District AIDS Council. A map of the province flashed from the projector onto the white screen at the front of the room in *Bairro Natite's* training center for health workers. Color coded, the key at the bottom indicated the government's reliance on foreign aid, and it's supposed supervisory role. Districts were divided between several international initiatives (including some PEPFAR contractors) and smaller actors such as humanitarian NGOs (e.g., Medicos del Mundo). "But," Manuel continued, "this won't be possible for us, from a logistical perspective. It's only from the level of coordination that it can happen. That's why you're all here."

He gazed at the audience, composed of thirty people, mostly program directors and AIDS activists, volunteers of home-based care programs throughout the province. "I want you all to know that at the Núcleo, we are working in a political box. Things are being decided in Maputo over which we have no control. In particular, activists are supposed now to work across all health areas, not just HIV. Things are changing. We don't know where they are going." As Manuel stepped aside to speak to a Spanish man seated at the front of the room, I turned to Carlitos. "Do you know what he's talking about?" I asked. Carlitos shrugged his shoulders.

Manuel continued, "Since last year, in Maputo, we haven't been able to settle the issue of incentives for activists doing home-based care. It seems like nobody can decide whether providing them is a good idea or not. Some say it's not fair. In some cases, two NGOs are working in the same place, and one person is working for both NGOs, taking home a double salary. In other cases, some NGOs pay better than others. People leave one NGO and go to work for another only for the money. People get trained and then disappear." At this, the coordinator for Medicos del Mundo, the Spanish man, stood to comment:

> This is the problem we find across the board, and often, we can't even verify if the work is getting done. It's not just with the activists that we already have. We tried to train twenty-five traditional birth attendants in Metuge, but from day one, they wanted to get paid, so they abandoned the training. Many even refused to take an HIV test. We can train them and give them tools, but they shouldn't be doing

that kind of work if they are HIV positive. What we've found is that the easiest thing is just to pay for these women to attend school. (Toni, international NGO coordinator)

Toni continued to speak on the problems associated with activists—they're untrustworthy, don't report for work, and often demand more money after they're hired. The organization was leaning toward disbanding their team of activists entirely. "The problem with doing that," he said, "is that we have no other way now of knowing which HIV patients are still taking their medications and which have stopped. We used to get the register from the hospital for this, but not anymore."

The meeting continued with presentations from other coordinators of home-based care programs. The coordinator from AMODEFA—the Mozambican Association for the Defense of the Family—said they trained seventy-four activists in Nangade, Palma, and Mueda, focusing especially on adherence concerns. "One of the things that we have them do," said the AMODEFA coordinator, "is go door-to-door to those homes where we suspect the patient hasn't been to the hospital in some time. It's guesswork, primarily." He showed his own PowerPoint slide, a map of the town of Palma, with some areas shaded out. "Just months after the training, we lost half of our activists in Palma because of the issue of payment, leaving these few locations [pointing at the map] where the program continues."

He cited the additional barrier of long distances and infrequent transport, leading the remaining activists to spend more time walking between homes than working with patients. "We're guessing that almost half of patients who start treatment don't go back after the first month. This is what we are trying to attack." He began to list the names of organizations that provided funding support. "It's not enough . . . [turning to face Manuel] there's really no way we can expand the program in this situation as it is."

The last NGO to present the results of its home-based care program, the Spanish NGO Medicus Mundi, working in the district of Montepuez, had the clearest data on the subject: "We have 173 beneficiaries. Half of them are HIV positive, some of these and another 10 percent suffer from psychiatric disorders, such as schizophrenia and depression. There are a lot of alcoholics. We've dedicated a small room in the hospital to these psychiatric and substance abuse patients and have begun to treat them" (Isabel, nurse and international NGO coordinator). The coordinator, Isabel, mentioned that turnover in the program was high. There were a lot of deaths. Others disappeared, probably going to other villages or towns. She continued, "We have eighty-two new patients just this month, so there is a continuing need. We have only thirty-four patients on ART, and five of them abandoned their medications last month. We know this is not good and are working hard to educate people about this." After the meeting and her discussion, I approached Isabel about her statistics, and she invited me to spend some time with her and the NGO's activists in Montepuez.

About two hundred kilometers from Pemba, Montepuez is not densely populated. The entire district is inhabited by an estimated 187,000 persons, but it had the second highest HIV prevalence in the province, just after Pemba City, at about 8 percent. Isabel knew of my interest in gauging the number of *abandonos*, or those on ART but lost to follow-up. She told me that "the hospital officially records zero of these cases, but our records indicate it is much more than that because only about two-thirds of the patients actually come to pick up their medications every month." Riding through the town of Montepuez on my first morning with her, she had to stop the Landcruiser on three separate occasions because somebody was walking or lying in the middle of the street. The activists in the car with us recognized each of them as HIV patients, each time descending to query the individual and either point them in the right direction, accompany them home, or take them to the hospital.

After delicately chaperoning one of these people into the back of the car where I was seated, an activist told me that "this woman is on phenobarbitol and haloperidol"—antipsychotic medications—and "when we first found her, her family had left her at the *curandeiro*'s [traditional healer's compound], where she tested negative for *majinni* [evil spirits]." I glanced at the woman, who was wearing a white but extremely dirty full wedding dress. She mumbled occasionally as we got closer to the hospital. "She stays alone?" I asked.

"She moves around," replied the activist. "We never know where she might show up!"

Medicus Mundi had twenty activists on the payroll who carried out home-based care duties in each section of town. As we dropped the woman in the wedding dress and her activist guide at the hospital, we encountered Bento, one of the male activists, waiting for us outside. He had encountered trouble that morning getting a patient to be seen by one of the doctors, and the man remained collapsed on a reed mat outside of the entrance, having waited all night for the place to open. Isabel told me that in her opinion, "the female activists really work much better. But Bento is very good. The problem with the women is that sometimes their husbands forbid them from working. We train them and then they're gone after a month." I waited as Isabel went to talk to one of the hospital staff. I noticed she had to raise her voice, but then, someone came out to fetch the man on the reed mat. After this, together with Bento, we entered the Landcruiser again to start the day's rounds. Isabel was going to introduce me to some of the beneficiaries of the home-based care program.

Just off the main streets of Montepuez, there are neighborhoods with many homes that are on neither the electrical nor the water grid. In these cases, other than proximity to certain services or businesses, the residents may as well be located in rural villages. We parked the vehicle in the yard of a home constructed in the pique-no-pão style—a bamboo frame with rocks packed in between to form walls and a mud layer covering them to provide a finished look and seal the cracks. It was thatching season. Nearby lay a pile of grass destined for that purpose, tied neatly in large bundles and stacked into a pyramid shape. An older woman came out to greet us; I could barely see anything in the dark interior of the home as she shut the door behind her. After exchanging pleasantries with Bento in Makua, she went back inside and came out again with a small girl, maybe six or seven years old, in her arms. "This is the patient," said Bento. "We have known her for about four months." The girl had just woken up but smiled widely, extending her hand to shake mine and Isabel's. "Her mother and father are dead, so her grandmother here takes care of her," he said. He pointed inside the house and the girl went back in, emerging quickly with a large envelope and a pill bottle.

Spilling the pills onto a tray he began to count them—triomune, a common fixed-dose ARV tablet—while the girl pulled what turned out to be an X-ray from the envelope. "She also had tuberculosis, but it's clear now," said Isabel, holding the X-ray up against the whitewashed backdrop of the house's mud wall. She motioned for the girl to pull off the head scarf she was wearing, revealing patchy skin and not very much hair. The girl herself hadn't spoken, and I was beginning to pick up on the fact that she was deaf. "What happened to her hearing?" I asked.

Bento responded, "When she was very little she was treated for malaria with quinine. Deafness sometimes results. There is another boy inside, also with TB, and we think he is positive also, but the grandmother here doesn't trust Isabel and won't let us treat the boy. She said that she doesn't want a white woman telling her how to take care of the child and that the hospital hasn't done well with the other one. We haven't been able to get him tested."

The next home we went to was a government constructed one, with cement blocks, glass windows, and asbestos roofing. We circled around to the backyard. The patient's husband, a former civil servant, had died, and she lived alone. On her arms were spotty, red, and irregularly shaped fungal lesions—mycosis. Bento pulled a vial of medicine from his bag, and we waited as he used a cotton swab to paint her tongue with a purple liquid, an antiseptic, intended to help treat the candidiasis that covered the inside of her mouth. As she sat down, Isabel began to question her. "We heard you were having some problems, what happened?" In Portuguese, the woman began to explain that her allergies were very bad, and the worst one was her allergy to water. She couldn't take a bath because of it. "You're not bathing?" asked Isabel. The woman shook her head and told us that she didn't have any soap.

Seeing us, a neighbor shouted something to Bento in Makua. "I think she's been robbed," he said. At this, the patient became more animated and explained that a robber had entered her house as she slept, stealing her food (maize flour), cooking pans, and a blanket. Isabel became visibly angry. "We've talked about this before!" She stood up and began pacing. "Every time you get something, it's gone the next day. You can't keep track of your [health] papers, and now you're not even bathing. I'm not even sure that you want to be our patient. . . . Do you want to be our patient?" The woman nodded yes.

Isabel continued, "Then you have to take responsibility for your own health, you have to bathe . . . OK?" Again, the woman nodded yes. She was also suffering from a pink eye infection, and so Isabel donned a pair of rubber gloves and asked the woman to lie down on the reed mat where she was sitting. To keep the woman from fighting, Bento held her arms to her side, as Isabel held her eyes open and inserted eye drops. Isabel, clearly frazzled, stood up and poured water from a jug into a shallow pan. At this, the patient broke Bento's grip, rose to her feet, and moved quickly toward her house. She entered and slammed the door, leaving us all shocked and ready to leave. As we went back to the car, Isabel explained to me that the woman had worsening HIV-related dementia. "I don't know how long we can keep doing this with her . . . it's terrible. I don't know if she can stay in our program, our level of care isn't high enough, and she needs somebody with her all of the time."

The next place we stopped was the local Assembly of God church, close to the center of town. We didn't go in but went around to the side of the building, where a tarpaulin had been erected. A man was roasting cassava and boiling a small pot of water over a fire. "This man is positive, but also is an epileptic," Bento explained to me as we greeted him. He told me that his name was Vasilio, and he came here from Mesa, about thirty kilometers away. He wanted to go back, but his daughter and her new husband had kicked him out of their home. His wife had done the same thing a few months earlier and now he was homeless. "They let me sleep here, in the church," he said, "but they still haven't given me a bed. I have to sleep on the floor." He explained that he got some food from a government program for HIV patients, "but it's not enough."

As Bento counted the man's pills and filled out the home-based care form, Isabel stepped away from us to attend to a phone call. At that point, among men only, Vasilio explained even more of his story—that he was impotent and his wife left him for that reason, leading eventually to their separation and his current lack of family. After we left him with his cooking fire, Isabel and I discussed the man's needs. In our own countries—the United States or Spain—the government cannot subsidize everyone who needs food or housing, and we have our own homeless populations. How is it possible that Mozambicans expect this in their own nation, with even fewer resources? Vasilio's story, hardly unique, was nevertheless common in his insistence that he'd be even better housed and fed than with what was currently provided.

At our next stop, the patient had been given her own room—outside of the family's house, in the backyard, in what looked to be a simple and unwelcoming storage space. Upon entering the compound, the family barely greeted us, stayed seated, and kept shelling peas. Noticing our arrival, the female patient came outside for what was probably the first time that day, looking sleepy or groggy. The family—her sisters, cousins, and children—ignored her; they seemed to want nothing to do with her. Her left eye was swollen, and Isabel sat down to have a closer look. The patient had recently recovered from measles. Speaking Makua, with Bento translating, the woman told us that some man had broken into her room last night and had sex with her. She was tossed off her mat, and her pillow was thrown to the other side of the room. "She says it was an evil spirit," said Bento. Complaining of stomach aches, Isabel asked how she was taking the anti-inflammatory that she had been given. "She's taking too many of them," Bento told us. While that probably accounted for the stomach ache, the woman insisted that she had a cobra inside of her and when it moved it caused her pain.

Glancing inside the room, Isabel asked her why she wasn't using her mosquito net. She told us it was because there are no mosquitoes this time of year, but when Bento asked her to show us the net, it was still inside its original packaging. During the visit, the family continued to ignore our conversation, avoided eye contact, and acted as if we weren't there. Close to her family, yet separated from the home, it wasn't clear if the woman was even getting enough to eat. She appeared skinny for a patient who was actively on treatment. Isabel asked for her health card, to see if she was attending the day hospital and picking up her medication on time, but the women told us that she didn't have either—her card or her medications—because her usual visiting activist (not Bento)—had stolen them.

As we departed from that home, Isabel and Bento told me about Ricardo, an activist who had worked with the program for some time but then disappeared. During his tenure, he gained the trust of Medicus Mundi and the patients he served through near-perfect attendance at meetings, in the clinic, and at appointments at patient's homes. By the time Isabel started hearing negative comments from other activists about him, he had already caused a lot of damage. Because he filled out fake reports, Medicus Mundi was unaware that his visits were less frequent than they should have been. He also violated protocol by keeping the patient's health cards and medications on his person or in his own home, allegedly in order to sell the medications to sellers in the local market.

In Pemba, I had seen in the markets tables stocked with HIV medications, even entire bottles with the Ministry of Health logo on the front. Talking with the sellers, I knew that some people did access treatment in this manner, even buying one or two pills at a time. Given the educational level of many patients in Montepuez, and their incapacity to care for themselves, Ricardo's affront was a serious one. In many cases, people depended on activists to provide accurate information and guidance on what to do in certain situations, how and when to take medication, and what events should trigger a visit to the clinic. The last patient that we visited was not alone in having her health card and medications go missing; Ricardo was in charge of nine or ten other patients who had also not been well attended to in recent times.

In Montepuez, *ordinary people* did not benefit as well as expected from being enrolled in Cabo Delgado's most sophisticated home-based care program. Though Medicus Mundi and activists working for the NGO possessed most of the needed elements for success—medication, transport, scientific knowledge and authority—common ground was missing, compromising the NGO's efforts and patients' ability to comply: a grandmother who didn't trust a white nurse with a sick child, a woman with worsening dementia and a debilitating "allergy" to water, a man demanding resources much greater than his government or a local church could give him, a woman claiming to be under supernatural attack and a family that treated her as if she was already dead. The socially constructed "realities" of people in Montepuez, because they were able to impose themselves upon the NGO's plans, cannot be simply dismissed. In the right context, they are intelligible and comprehensible.

These misunderstandings point to alternative worldviews crafted, in part, by uneven access to information. The fix for this dilemma is not simply more pills, clinics, health care staff, or food rations but rather better mediators—persons and opportunities to help reconcile the different realities and knowledges that circulate in Montepuez and places like it. Put differently, incomplete or unsuccessful *socialization* may account for the heterogeneity in people's attitudes and circumstances, limiting the efficacy of official programs and their relevance in the lives of *ordinary people*.

Logically, it follows that good local activism and support groups could help remedy the situation, but we see also—in Ricardo—the example of an activist who subverted the NGO's program and took advantage of vulnerable patients. While this problem arose most obviously from poor NGO oversight, it could occur just as easily in any hierarchical arrangement. Before I left Montepuez, I questioned Isabel about whether the government would eventually take over Medicus Mundi's programs. She explained that the government viewed the home-based care program as an NGO initiative and chose to remain uninvolved. If the NGO were to leave, the program would likely stop. Because Montepuez had no AIDS association or support groups, many of the activists carrying out home-based care were not HIV-positive; rather, they were appointed by the *presidentes dos bairros* (neighborhood presidents) and were most often the friends or relatives of local political elites and upper-middle-class families. If the state took on the program, it might even deteriorate.

When incentives are tied to the role of caregiver, and responsibilities for others doled out according to status and privilege rather than merit or a record of good service, no matter who's in charge, the potential for predatory behavior is always there. Isabel, an expatriate and the sole coordinator of the program, lamented the lack of a local AIDS association able to help her with this aspect of the job but did not want to create one herself for fear it would not be sustainable. Based on these encounters in Montepuez, the challenge for AIDS activists the world over is how to inspire appropriate exchanges and sensibilities in places like this while avoiding the pitfalls of payment, funding, and outsider control or supervision.

TREATMENT ILLITERACY AND ABANDONMENT

It is easier to enroll patients in treatment programs than it is to retain them. Over the past decade, the number of new ART patients in Cabo Delgado Province rose from 5,500 people (in 2008) to just more than 9,000 (in 2013) and to almost 21,000 (in 2016; MISAU 2017b). These numbers are consistently higher than expected goals, amounting to about 130 percent of projected new enrollees. As time goes on, however, patients drop out of the system. Typically, retention is measured at the one-, two-, and three-year marks. National averages estimate patient retention in Mozambique at 70 percent (year 1), 52 percent (year 2), and 49 percent (year 3). Averages are a little lower in Cabo Delgado, at about 63 percent (year 1), 42 percent (year 2), and 40 percent (year 3). As global efforts to place patients on ART unfold faster and more widely than ever before, retention in Cabo Delgado is getting worse instead of better, dropping 16 percentage points since 2013 (from 56 to 40 percent) for patients on ART for three years. Combating poor patient retention requires addressing patients' desires and their ability to adhere to the prescribed pharmaceutical regimen. This turns out to be not so simple and may require more thought and innovation than many global health authorities can deliver.

The most commonly cited reasons for poor treatment adherence include distances to facilities, money for transportation, bad patient counseling, and drug availability (Groh et al. 2011). Adherence is also a psychological struggle, having much less to do with clinic access than often presumed. While this is increasingly recognized (Ware et al. 2009), these "psychological" barriers are harder to target—or to predict and "fix"—than standard, clinical ones. Some people stop taking the pills because they feel healthy and believe they are cured. Others stop for the opposite reason, because they feel unhealthy and believe the pills are making their condition worse. Some are hiding their HIV status and fear the discovery of pills by others in the home, being seen picking them up at the pharmacy, or making frequent visits to the hospital.

Other factors may break down a patient's resolve to be compliant. Side effects can be persistent and include nausea, vomiting, fatigue, diarrhea, headaches, constipation, loss of appetite, insomnia, and anxiety. Patients who are not well counseled may try to minimize uncomfortable side effects by voluntarily interrupting treatment, but in doing so, they compromise their immunological status and recovery in the process. Adherence is also not easy to measure. Some laboratory tests can do this—blood reference ranges, viral load, and CD4+ T-cell counts can provide reliable assessments—but the most common way to gauge patient compliance is by counting the number of pills left over in the pill bottle. Adherence, therefore, is usually self-reported (Denison et al. 2015; Simoni et al. 2006), and poor adherence is higher in some subgroups compared to others. The risk factors most frequently associated with poor adherence include unemployment, low income, low education, substance abuse, younger age, and an unstable home environment (Heath et al. 2002; Norton et al. 2010).

In Cabo Delgado, an important contribution to ensure patient adherence is for the family or caregiver to be aware that the patient has HIV and to know how the treatment works. HIV is seen as a new disease and different from many others because it is chronic and incurable. This poses an obstacle for people unaccustomed to being on medication for extended periods of time:

I have this epidemic [meaning HIV/AIDS]. And it is not like malaria, it doesn't go away, ever. I can't get my family to understand this, and so, the medication itself is not the same either. If you have TB, they give you pills for a certain time period and tell you that when you have taken them all, then you can stop. This virus is so different. We can't stop the pills! My mother doesn't believe that I can't just get an injection and stop the [hospital] visits. I tell her that with ART, the bugs that are inside my body stop moving and rest instead but never die, and this is the only way to keep them from killing me. I tell her that I am always sick, so I must keep going to the hospital. That is what sick people do, right? (Salima, ART patient)

Activists believe family involvement is lacking but essential to keep patients healthy and enrolled in programs:

When we are visiting the homes of patients, we find families that tell us the patient is already dead, when they are not. The patient is just in recovery, but it's not clear to them what is happening. They don't even know the name of the illness that the patient is suffering from. They just see reactions [from the pills] and say, "Ah, these medications are not good!" They see vomiting, and maybe the patient is acting silly from being light-headed, or the legs are itching. It doesn't matter how many times you counsel them, or the patient; you can talk to them one thousand times, but until they see the improvement themselves, it doesn't make any difference. These cases are just complicated. (focus group, Moçimboa da Praia hospital)

At the worst, families may even discourage treatment and be involved in keeping patients off medication:

Here [in Macomia], the family is usually responsible for making people stop their medication. They complain about the price of transport. They tell us that since we feel better, it's time to quit taking the pills. I could have listened to my aunt, but instead, I went on my own. These are the same people who told me not even to get a test, that the needles they use are the same ones that gave me the virus, even the cotton they put on your finger is infected, or that the blood they have taken out of others is just passed on to you. They will even tell you that the medications themselves cause AIDS. (focus group, Macomia)

These types of statements reinforce what many researchers have already acknowledged, that families and caregivers—particularly when they can help make sure that patients take their medication—should be included in HIV/AIDS programs (Walton et al. 2004). Western understandings of confidentiality may inhibit this at the village level.

Such mistrust of biomedicine is common in Cabo Delgado. The hospital and the clinic are relatively recent historical introductions to Mozambique and to the province (Bastos 2007). Some people believe that health facilities are under the control of foreigners and white colonizers and that doctors and nurses intentionally give illnesses to patients in order to control the population. Health care workers are, according to some of my interviewees, "donos de doenca" (the owners of disease), tricksters who seek to harm people, destroy families, and fragment society by spreading diseases. For some patients, even visiting the hospital is a psychological battle: "For me, I have no problem going to the hospital because my father, when I was a child, worked for whites and always told me that it was OK to do that. Others don't think so. My friend still thinks that the nurses here are tricking him, that the reason the government is giving away medicine is because it is a government project" (Bonifacio, ART patient). Some ART patients are quick to try to end their relationship with the clinic and do so as soon as they begin to recover: "When you go to the hospital you find good things, not bad ones. I didn't know this before! So when some people get tested and get their [HIV/AIDS health] card and their medications and they start to feel better, they return to the hospital and try to hand the card back to the nurses. They tell them, 'Here is your card back; I don't need it anymore'" (Acácio, ART patient). On other accounts, patients insist that they have, on occasion, been given the wrong kind of medicines or medicines that don't really work. In some cases, concerns about the integrity of health care staff are warranted. Some health workers "go rogue" and operate personal businesses out of their homes:

> A nurse who was here [at Pemba's hospital] used to treat patients in his own home. You could pay him less, and instead of waiting in line, it was faster. He used to give injections of aspirin. While he had a lot of customers, it was later we found out he did not know what he was doing and that he stole supplies from the hospital for this business. [I ask her why people went to see him at all.] Because he would tell you what is wrong with you and give personal advice, while in the hospital, you just got pills. If you were very sick, you could sleep in his home. (Lesley, ART patient)

Treatment literacy in this area trends very low. Few patients were able to name their medications, and they tended to describe them instead by their color—white, brown, pink, and so on. When asked what ARVs they were taking, occasionally someone would pull out their clinic health card and let me read the name of the medication written there.

A common misconception about AIDS activism is that it helps patients feel a sense of ownership over their own health care and pharmaceutical regimen. In Pemba, the government, rather than AIDS activists, gets credit for providing drugs to patients, who feel indebted as a result and possibly even insecure about the future of their treatment. "Please don't stop bringing these medications here! My health is guarded there in these pills. I started taking them so that I could be a human being again! So I am glad that people have arranged this, when we, the patients, weren't even thinking about it. They will decide what to do next. [I asked her who she was referring to.] Our government and people like you" (Sheron, ART patient).

ART patients are not always able to cope with the side effects of their medications. These range from constant hunger (the most common complaint), to peripheral neuropathy (such as loss of sensation in the feet), to an overwhelming feeling approximating drunkenness or intoxication, to even a loss of eyesight or blurred vision. Certain rashes, sometimes painful, itchy, or ugly, come and go as they please. For many patients, "the reaction to the medication is very bad, and some people abandon them because they are afraid to die and think that the pills will kill them before the virus does." It's a shock, to some, to find out that what is supposed to make one feel better has the opposite immediate effect and being told by the provider that side effects will wear off doesn't make the experience any easier to tolerate.

AIDS associations and informal support groups are important for patients to work through some of these issues. When they can meet together, patients recognize that they are not alone:

> I used to forget at first [to take the pills], but I'm very well accustomed now. I used to vomit all of the time because I had a lot of saliva in my mouth and my throat. Now I can't see very well. I think that is because of the pills. My left arm has no strength, so I come here [to the day hospital] for massages twice a week. I also have trouble reading—and that's not just because of my eyes, it's like I can't think sometimes; I feel a little stupid, like my brain can't function. I know this is caused by the treatment because others [in the association] have the same problem. (Miguel, AIDS association member)

The relationship between ART and the body is summarized most frequently in statements about insufficient amounts or varieties of food worsening the experience. Many discussed the fact that when unable to eat at medication time, they felt "drunk" and suffered more intense reactions and side effects than when taking medications on a full stomach. Many refused to take pills without food as a result. The uncomfortable nature of side effects, and their clear relationship to the medication itself, is an abrogating factor to adherence, particularly for patients who have not suffered more intense symptoms and may be tempted to quit because they haven't yet experienced what happens when they do.

Many patients credit that kind of personal experience—a frightening and near deadly disease episode or relapse—as the reason they are able to maintain adherence to ARVs later on. Making a clear connection between treatment and health assists in their personal resolve:

> The first fourteen days are very tough. If you aren't well educated, you can believe that you are cured within one week. There is a lack of information about this, and those of us who join associations are easier to help. Otherwise, you just don't know where some of these people live. It's easy to talk yourself out of coming back to the hospital. You've just found out you have this virus, it costs money to take transport, and you start to think that the government doesn't know what they are talking about [concerning treatment for life] because you feel great! Look, the nurses don't have the thirty minutes to do proper counseling in the hospital, so the biggest problem is starting the medications when you don't even think you have a serious illness. For me, I was so sick when they found me that I knew ARVs saved my life, *sem duvida* [no doubt]. (Carlos, AIDS association vice-president)

When I started ART in 2006, I got much better, and quickly. I was playing football and was very healthy. I was given two months' worth of the pills, but I only took a few of them. I put them on my shelf and left them there, started drinking again, and in a few weeks ended up with TB and so sick I couldn't leave the bed, again. Now, I would never abandon these medications, and I don't drink. The others in my association [he is the vice-president] look to me on this issue, so when someone wants to stop, I go and talk to them. [I ask him if that helps people continue.] In most cases, yes, but we have one or two who keep dropping out [of treatment]. (Crispen, AIDS association member)

One such example—of association members stopping treatment—was Eliza, a member of the association Nashukuru who showed up for an interview with me in Mecufi. When I asked her about her own adherence to medication, she told me she never questioned the efficacy of the medications and never quit taking them. My standard questions about side effects, stigma, and other challenges to her compliance didn't inspire any discussion. However, in later interviews with other association members, her name was often mentioned. I was told by several other members of her association that she was stubbornly nonadherent, that they had to keep watch over her daily to try to keep her on schedule. On three separate occasions, she was admitted to the hospital because she quit taking her pills and had not told anyone. Each time, her health deteriorated to a level more threatening and dangerous than before.

When I asked these other association members why she let this happen, nobody could tell me. She lived alone, her children had left the area, and she had no husband. She also had no income and no regular way to obtain food. Other association members had to bring her meals. The woman did not care for her own hygiene and rarely bathed. Others in the village accused her of being a witch and treated her as an outcast. Even though her trips to the clinic after she had ceased treatment restored her to health each time, she continued to falter and miss doses. Her reasons for this may be complicated. Perhaps, regardless of her experiences in the clinic, she did not believe she was HIV positive. Or perhaps she had no reason to live. Socially abandoned, reliant only on others in her AIDS association, she spent her days isolated or depressed, which did not help her poor adherence.

In a similar way, one Caridade activist, Reggie, insisted to me that he never stopped taking his medications. However, when he was away from the group, people talked about his noncompliant behavior. Reggie was newly married to a woman who, as far as we knew, was not HIV positive. She was considered overbearing, mean-spirited, and difficult to deal with. In spite of being an active member of Caridade and a vocal participant in meetings, Reggie had not told her, his third wife, about his own HIV-positive status. The two fought constantly. His neighbor, also a Caridade member, related these incidents. Plates and food would fly across the yard at mealtimes. Loud shouts could be heard from the bedroom at night.

Reggie's movements were monitored intensely because his wife feared he had other lovers. Reggie lied to his wife about the nature of Caridade, telling her that it was a Frelimo political party association. He also had to visit the day hospital unnoticed and kept his pills hidden. The result of this was more than just an occasional missed dose. At times, he handed over his pill bottle to his neighbor (also an association member), asking him to hide it so that his wife wouldn't find out his secret. He went days at a time without asking for his medication back, skipping doses because of this domestic situation.

When, one day, he finally was caught taking pills by his wife, he told her that he had a headache and that the pills were Tylenol rather than ARVs. Fortunately, Reggie never suffered a disease relapse. His noncompliant behavior probably wouldn't have stopped. One day, however, his wife showed up at the Caridade office looking for him. With a triomune thirty-pill bottle in her hand, which she claimed to have found in their latrine, she told the group present at the time that she finally knew they were all HIV positive. From that point, she tried to prohibit Reggie from participating in Caridade meetings and from taking his pills. The relationship ended in divorce. Reggie remained in Caridade, but he was transferred to live and work in a distant village for his own protection. When I saw him months later, he was healthier looking and told me he was much happier working at his new post.

Another Caridade activist, Armando, stopped taking ARVs because the clinic in his home village refused him service. When he was diagnosed in Pemba, he was given several months of medication. But when he arrived home, he found that his patient file had not been transferred. When his prescription ran out, the clinic refused to give him medications because his CD4+ cell count was above average. The workers there did not want to enroll him in their ARV program until he met the requirements of less than five hundred cells/mm^3. They did not believe Armando, who claimed that he had already initiated treatment in Pemba and just ran out of medication. He was told he would have to go back to Pemba and find his patient file before they would administer ARVs to him.

Unable to pay for transport back to Pemba, Armando stayed home. After several months off treatment, his condition began to deteriorate, and he came close to death. His neighbors and other villagers became aware of his HIV-positive status. At the insistence of activists working for an NGO there, Armando was driven to Pemba and nursed back to health in the hospital. As a result of everyone knowing his HIV-positive status, he did not feel safe or welcome in his home village. He joined Caridade and stayed in Pemba, and was trained as an activist. He eventually began to work and got paid for coordinating other activists in Caridade programs. Armando's story is, on one hand, unique. Most patients who want to be on treatment can usually obtain it from the clinic, but this is not always the case. Bureaucratic inefficiency and miscommunication pose legitimate threats to patients when protocols change or standards are too inflexible to take special cases into consideration.

Even living near to a clinic—where patients are more likely to have ready access to drugs—does not guarantee high treatment adherence. Clinical data as well as home-based care visits in Pemba and Montepuez, cities that had day hospitals close to patient homes, reveal that treatment abandonment is just as bad, if not worse, in urban areas compared to rural ones. Patient travel is likely not the most significant obstacle to treatment adherence. It is not at all unusual to find patients in the middle of urban *bairro* enrolled in an ART program who, when asked why they weren't taking their pills, simply shrug their shoulders and provide no answer. Even the best efforts of a local volunteer, one who lives in the same neighborhood and speaks the same language as the nonadherent patient, fails to convince him or her that the pills are lifesaving, that the hospital offers the best treatment compared to any other option that might be pursued—usually alternative means like traditional healing or prayer.

A simple or mundane excuse is sometimes all that's necessary to rationalize one's way out of medical treatment—the health care staff isn't friendly, the patient no longer gets free food rations, pills are not well tolerated, or the patient feels better—these are all easy ways for people to lose heart in biomedical treatment. On multiple occasions, I found myself without a response to those patients most socially isolated and most forlorn when they said that the pills make them hungry, that they can't afford anything to eat, and that they preferred to just die now rather than later (Kalofonos 2010).

One case that was particularly striking involved a woman with a six-month-old baby, who moved to Pemba seeking to become employed as a cleaning maid for a wealthy household. Her husband had abandoned her and the baby, and after leaving her village, she found herself living in a decrepit hut a five-minute walk away from the provincial hospital. When we arrived at her home during a home-based care visit, her pill bottle was empty. She asked me to buy a candle for her. This woman—who spent her nights in a dark home while the city around her teemed with electricity, loud music, parties, buses, and cars and minutes away from an international airport where tourists arrive, ready to spend U.S.$1,000 per night staying at nearby luxury island resorts—had no light, no matches, no food, and no help from her neighbors. She became distraught during our visit with her, as the activists asked questions about her health and welfare.

Holding her newborn baby by the wrist like a ragdoll, she insisted that their lives were worthless and threatened to kill herself that night. She was literally dragged the kilometer uphill to the hospital, where she received a thorough scolding from a worker in a hospital uniform who forced her medications down her throat. Distance did not threaten this woman. Had the hospital been any closer, it would only have been a little bit more tolerable for the activists to drag her there. More invested in projects than patients, the local AIDS associations could not offer much help in the form of a well-functioning support group—no food, money, or even practical advice. This situation was not at all unusual.

Anthropologists studying these phenomena—patient noncompliance, resistance to taking medication, and poor treatment adherence—place them in the category of biomedical skepticism and question whether it is even possible to address this in the context of the clinic. The social factors of poor treatment adherence—overcoming stigma, persevering through difficult cycles of side effects, combating fatalism, or not trusting authority—are considered problems unsolvable given only the brief periods of patient-provider interaction (Moyer and Hardon 2014; Hardon and Moyer 2014). Like Eliza, some patients may simply tell the provider that they are compliant when they are not. This has been documented as very likely in situations where medicines, such as ARVs, are not cures but only treatments, temporary, in constant need of replacement.

Studying the use of benzodiazepines (Smith and Tett 2010; Britten 1996), scholars note dissatisfaction among patients who feel that the drugs do not address the root causes of their anxiety and thus refuse their medications. Studying the use of Antabuse (Steffen 2005), a drug used to make heavy drinkers sick so that they cannot continue to drink, some research equates refusal to take the pills with disobedience to authority. Studying people with epilepsy (Mbuba et al. 2012; Conrad 1985), researchers point out that some patients associate the drugs with the illness and assume, incorrectly, that by not taking the drugs their illness will fade or go away. Others note how daily routines and work necessary for survival can take precedence over adherence, especially when physical labor—as in African subsistence farming—is negatively impacted by side effects (Trostle 1988; Alcano 2009). In other cases, patients stop taking pills after a certain period of time because it is a habit that they have not routinized or chosen to maintain (Winchester et al. 2017).

The most common reason for HIV treatment abandonment in Cabo Delgado approximates what soldiers experience from overexposure to combat, war, and death. Most patients who stop their treatment, or are tempted to do so, go through a personalized version of "combat fatigue" (Jones 2006). Struggling with their own negative and destructive thoughts and actions, or with others in their same household or society, several factors contribute to a breakdown in the psyche—a stress disorder or a response to anxiety, fear, and hopelessness. The way to engage this is by developing strength and resilience in all aspects of life—at work, at home, and at play (Frankl 2006)—to keep this from taking such a toll on the patient's willpower and resolve to keep living and fighting the persistent battles necessary to keep the virus at bay.

From visits to clinics and hospitals all over Cabo Delgado, it is obvious that treatment abandonment is a serious concern in the province. In the rooms where patient files are kept, stacks of them are set aside and marked in red with the word *abandonado* (defaulter) across the front. The responsibility of tracking down these patients is not usually a government task. Rather, volunteer activists have the difficult assignment of finding the patient at home and recording their status in official log books. If the patient is deceased, he or she will be removed from the registry. If not, the activist attempts to link the patient with services again, bring the patient in to the hospital for reevaluation, or continue to visit the patient—possibly taking medications to them in the interim, if clinicians are willing to bend the rules—until the patient agrees to be seen again by health care staff at the facility. It is a difficult job, and some NGOs hire staff and coordinators specifically for this task. They are always overworked because the number of patients who do not report back to the clinic is overwhelming and never seems to go down.

Good adherence is a function of determination. Those patients who are most successful have others encouraging them and providing "social capital" for maintaining their regimen (Binagwaho and Ratnayake 2009; Ware et al. 2009). What needs to be targeted—a patient's fortitude and capacity to maintain it via the moral and emotional support of those around them—is equally as important as drug availability and distribution at a point of service. Some programs and researchers have tried to incorporate methods for strengthening this in the clinical setting. These may involve the utilization of nonmedical help—like the use of "treatment supporters" (Kranzer and Ford 2011; Bärnighausen et al. 2011)—to provide a range of counseling services to patients.

These interventions fall into the category of "task shifting" policies (Bemelmans et al. 2010) intended to unburden doctors and nurses by devolving some duties to lower-level staff. But formalizing social support in this manner tends to be small scale and limited to a few select clinics or sites. The successes entailed, the results of initiatives carried out for evaluative purposes or as pilot projects, may be difficult to reproduce and not funded over the long term. The recommendations that come forth emphasize the need for tailoring services more to the lives of the patient, pinpointing barriers to adherence that impact them in their homes and various locales, educating them more thoroughly on the nature of ART, setting up reminders—via cell phones or mnemonic techniques—for patients to take their pills regularly and obtain refills when needed (Harries et al. 2010).

Surveying the literature on improving patient adherence, articles on this topic provide exhaustive but overly generalized recommendations that, quite likely, are too comprehensive, logistically challenging, or require more advanced resources for tasks like data management than is likely possible in most African contexts. Bärnighausen et al. (2011: 944) suggest the incorporation of "behavioural, cognitive, affective, and biological interventions through combinations of treatment supporters, nutritional support, financial support, psychosocial support, and education sessions." Brinkhof and colleagues (2010) recommend tracing patients lost to follow up in order to ascertain their vital status and more diligently recording transfers in and out of programs. In a recent document, the WHO (2013) prescribes addiction counseling, mental health support, and targeting services based on gender to address treatment program attrition. These kinds of questions—of how to provide services that cater to specific locales and for as many patients as possible—are really best addressed outside of the clinic rather than in it and by patients themselves.

But groups like Caridade, with conflict, infighting, and competition over resources, have not gone unnoticed. No small amount of frustration is felt by those in close contact with malfunctioning support groups. This has led to alternative efforts to get treatment to people, still in nontraditional ways, but doing away with those civil society elements that seem so problematic in favor of strictly ART-oriented services. Luque-Fernandez and colleagues (2013) discuss "adherence clubs" in South Africa. Facilitated by trained counselors, nurses visit with groups of fifteen to thirty patients who meet the inclusion criteria for participation, having been on ART for at least eighteen months. Basic health assessments are done during the meetings, and short discussions on HIV-related topics take place.

Decroo and colleagues (2014) discuss "Community ART Support Groups" in Mozambique—a model that is being increasingly embraced by the Ministry of Health—which involve groups of up to six members who verify one another's adherence and send a representative to the clinic to collect medication for the entire group. The representative relates important information to clinicians during the trip, which is documented on a shared group health card. Models like these have yielded substantially higher rates of adherence, generally more than 90 percent after a year or longer. If these types of initiatives become standard or more efficient than working with support groups, they might easily replace or compete with civil society projects and efforts in southern Africa.

In Cabo Delgado, as previously mentioned, about 60 percent of ART patients drop out of treatment programs after the three-year mark. That pharmaceutical adherence is so great a challenge for *ordinary people* there reflects not just the difficulties of clinic access but also how drug efficacy remains unestablished in the minds of most patients. Many patients, who do faithfully comply with their regimen, have suffered dramatically from prior symptomatic episodes. Some have bounced back from severe disease relapses and are able to make clear connections between their recovery and a commitment to the drugs. The catastrophic effects of going off ART can, ironically, serve as "proof" that HIV is a serious health threat and that treatment advocates are correct.

Biomedicine is not automatically given a high place of authority in southern Africa, and clinicians struggle to reach patients with this kind of information. What this means is that activists still have lots of work to do; there is ample evidence that people cannot simply be told to take their drugs by the health care staff and always successfully comply. There are obvious facets of lay psychology at work here that can be better transmitted and shared by and between patients in a support group rather than clinical setting. There is therefore a continuing need for nonclinical models and options for patients to sustain their treatment access and maintain the willpower or personal resolve required to stay on treatment.

ALCOHOLISM AND ART PATIENTS

It should come as no surprise that HIV-positive persons who regularly partake of alcohol suffer a higher risk of defaulting on treatment than those who do not (Huis In 't Veld et al. 2012). While this outcome may be reserved for those who drink to excess, in the southern African context, these are a majority over only social drinkers (WHO 2014). Moreover, beer and wine, the more expensive and less-intoxicating options, are not as frequently consumed or as readily available as hard liquor. Home-brewed spirits and uncontrolled brands of clear gin are ubiquitous.

That Mozambicans, even in the mostly Muslim north of the country, participate regularly in heavy episodic drinking is quite obvious, especially during the night. Moving through Pemba's *bairros* and alleyways, it is apparent that a considerable amount of drinking occurs when the sun is up as well. In general, heavy drinkers are 50 percent as likely to be classified as adherent to their treatment as nondrinkers, and missed doses of ARVs occur most often on drinking days (Hendershot et al. 2009). For some people in Caridade and other associations in the area, every day is a drinking day, and the question is not when to stop but how much can be obtained.

Of course, the official stance on mixing ARVs with alcohol is abstinence. During counseling sessions ART patients, particularly men, are warned against alcohol as a threat not only to adherence but to the efficacy of the pills as the body breaks them down chemically. However, there is no follow up to this information from the clinic. Unless a problem case emerges uncontested, someone with a drinking problem is unlikely to be confronted about it. Moreover, according to the published literature, interventions on this topic are scarce, or otherwise only brief and cursory in nature (Parry et al. 2014).

One of the biggest problems with this situation—the combination of telling patients to abstain with little guidance on how to manage this—is that patients may believe they must make a choice between the alcohol or the treatment

(Kalichman et al. 2013). Besides that, drinkers in general display overall sub-optimal adherence and higher mortality than other ART patients, making this topic one of increasing interest to those who work in the disease area of HIV and AIDS (Nachega et al. 2006). However, the attention being paid to alcohol abuse and ART is relatively new in the southern African context, which makes sense, because the effort to treat those with the virus has thus far focused on access and standard issues of recruitment and retention.

We have known since the start of the epidemic that substance abuse forms part of a wider web of risk-taking that, apart from the obvious (and even well studied) connection between intravenous drug use and HIV infection, places people at greater risk for contracting the virus through increased and danger-ous sexual activity (Needle et al. 1998). Alcohol use, though, compared to using dirty syringes for injecting drug use, isn't exactly some kind of outlier, unusual, or culturally unacceptable behavior in which to engage. Not only is alcohol popular and easy to obtain; it is marketed by national and international companies in a sophisticated manner (Casswell and Maxwell 2005). These include strategic product placement and other unmeasured promotions like sponsorships and point-of-sale materials. It is not unusual in Pemba to find people wearing free T-shirts distributed with the logo of 2M, the national beer. *Barracas* and other types of stores not only carry wide varieties of alcohol; some are also decked out with the brands and insignias of beer or dry gin companies, having received in-kind donations such as paint or signs with which to fix up the establishment.

In addition, during my stay, Pemba City only had five billboards—one near the airport, a couple in the center of town, and the other two near the beach—and four of them advertised alcohol like Johnny Walker Red Label Whiskey and Heineken Beer. The scenes depicted on these billboards highlight smiling faces, well-dressed but tightly clad women, or young men (next to their automobiles) enjoying one another's company with a drink in hand. These mar-keting tactics, however, are simply confirmation of a more obvious reality, that alcohol and drinking are at the confluence (and sometimes center) of many people's lives, as a vehicle for pleasure-seeking or entertainment during free time.

Alcohol also has its place in gender relations (Ray and Gold 1996), as a sign of masculinity or a proxy indicator for wealth that is meant to attract members of the opposite sex. Apart from being a drug in its own right, with the capacity to influence sexual decision-making, alcohol in southern Africa is also a basic and prolific cultural placeholder. In Pemba, this manifests most accessibly on the strand of Pemba (Wimbe) Beach, where tourists, politicians, business people, prostitutes, and many others mingle especially on Fridays and Sundays to wind down (or wind up) the week. Some take advantage of the opportunity by stock-ing up small coolers and selling individual beers, or sachets of gin or rum, by the roadside.

As night falls, the main drag along the beach becomes particularly attractive to partygoers. The expensive hotels and restaurants that normally stand out seem practically unimportant. The crumbling walls built during colonial Portuguese times, which separate the road from the start of the sand, are subsumed by and disappear behind the bodies of street hawkers and socializers as people sit, congregate, or display their wares on or by them. Cars parked alongside blast rhythms loud enough to spur impromptu dances. Meet-and-greets dominate the landscape, as people catch up with one another at the conclusion of the working week.

Besides alcohol, other things are sold here. Grilled chicken, samosas, cigarettes, and fruit, for example, are available. Women, their bodies for sale, are also on display in short shorts, tight T-shirts, and elaborate hairstyles. As the night progresses, so does the collective level of intoxication, and inhibitions drop. As the size of the crowd waxes, it becomes clear that for those who have the means—cars or motorcycles—the beach is the primary stop on a circuit of bars and restaurants that create a welcome escape and diversion from the drudgery of workaday life in the city.

Often, on Friday nights, I would sacrifice a full night's rest to absorb the goings on of nightlife on Pemba Beach. Sitting there along the wall, chatting with my neighbors, I see beach boys who frequented the area at all times of the day or night in order to prey on tourists (mostly by selling arts and crafts, other trinkets, or marijuana), and a dazzling array of vehicles stop and go along the strand. Some of them, mostly Landcruisers, are clearly emblazoned with the logo of the Republic of Mozambique. Others belong to USAID, or NGOs in the city headed by Mozambican national staff, such as Population Services International (an NGO that prides itself on HIV education and prevention, mostly through the distribution of condoms). Some vehicles belong to well-to-do residents, others to international businessmen on their way to or from Tanzania. The drivers of these vehicles stop, one person or all the people in the car get out, buy a beer or two, pick women to accompany them, then get back into the car and drive away. Motorcycles buzz back and forth as well, carrying on the routine. The same drivers sometimes reappear and repeat the process as the night goes on. The conversations between men and women as they barter on a fair price for sex can easily be overheard. The *quatorzinhas* (fourteen-year-old girls) are the most expensive.

On the other side of the wall, on the beach side, small groups of mostly local people sit in the sand, forming small circles, and engaging in lively conversation. Along the seashore, couples walk, sometimes hand-in-hand, sometimes smoking or drinking. It is not unusual to see groups of teenage or young adult boys loudly pursuing one attractive female. Sex on the beach is common at night. So are reports of gang rape. As the night drags on, fights often break out, and people haul each other into the nearby police station to settle what would otherwise be petty or resolvable arguments if alcohol were not involved. As the outdoor scene becomes increasingly anarchic, those who can afford it migrate into the discotheque at the end of the beach, remaining there until the sun comes up. Mozambicans—from Maputo to Cabo Delgado—know very well this practice of what can only be referred to as *uma festinha* (a little party). If one should move from the beach to the other bars or restaurants around the city, drinking (excessively) is the glue that holds the city together on the weekends—or tears it apart, depending on one's perspective.

Not to be outdone, those of lesser means, in the yards, housing compounds, and *barracas* of the bairros, also have their fill of alcoholic substances and partying. A stroll through any neighborhood reveals, especially on the corners of paths and unpaved roads less frequented by cars and trucks, brightly colored plastic buckets full of the yeast-heavy maize drink known as *cabanga*. This drink, less powerful than others, lends itself well to all-day drinking sessions and is particularly favored on national holidays when nobody works and for weddings or funerals. Often brewed by women trying to make money on the side, it takes at least a liter to even get a good buzz. Because the belly swells, locals claim that one need not eat when partaking of that much *cabanga*.

The opposite of this drink, the clear, distilled, corn-based moonshine known as *nipa*, ranges from 180- to 190-proof pure grain alcohol. For half a dollar, which buys about a half pint, one can become quite inebriated. For an entire dollar, or a whole pint, one can forget what happened for several hours. For those who buy in bulk, and for those who brew *nipa* themselves, the scene around the home can become not only sad or frightening but disastrous. The neighborhood of Chipapwale, the poorest and most inaccessible of Pemba's central bairros, is located on the opposite side of the bay from the beach, where the sewage and runoff water from the city gathers during flood times. As I was carrying out my research, Chipapwale was absolutely devastated by a *nipa* epidemic. Drunks literally crawled—even in broad daylight—from drinking spot to drinking spot, from one yard to another, in search of the substance they needed to stay inebriated.

I regularly interacted with and followed the lives of three Chipapwale residents who were also Caridade members—the treasurer, Fevereiro; the president, Antonio; and an activist named Rita. During my time with them, none of these people managed to escape the clutches of *nipa*. Fevereiro's girlfriend, his second after his divorce and a schoolteacher, once received a loan from the Agha Khan Foundation to fix up her home, a house that she shared with the treasurer. But rather than using the money for what it was intended, she bought supplies to manufacture *nipa* in their spare bedroom—a homemade contraption, a moonshine complete with pipes, glass jars, and a heating source. The children who slept there had to start sleeping in the sitting room. After her first batch, she got so drunk that she tried to pull down the electrical wires strung up through the rafters of their home, an effort to intentionally shock and kill herself.

Both of them addicted to *nipa*, the couple fought constantly. My visits there, subsequently, revealed the kinds of people that *nipa* attracts. At least one tried to sleep with Fevereiro's girlfriend while he was passed out drunk. Another stole their small television from inside of the house. Whenever I found people gathered there, half of them would be passed out, sometimes having soiled themselves, and would wake up occasionally for another drink. If payment was overdue and service was refused, voices were raised. The alcoholics would then move on, presumably to a location where one more shot or cup could be had.

Antonio, Caridade's president, lived just around the corner from Fevereiro. He had a wife and two children and used to own a number of expensive objects and furnishings. He had, over the course of several years, pawned his posses-sions, including refrigerators, televisions, and motorcycles when funding was too short for him to drink. Compared to others, Antonio was not that poor. As a nurse in the day hospital, he had a government salary. As the president of Caridade, he had some NGO money as well. Despite that, his children went around poorly clad and slept on reed mats instead of even the cheap, locally constructed sisal bedding that most families could afford. Whenever I visited, he begged money from me for a drink, and usually sent one of his children to a nearby *nipa* salesman to buy him a small bottle, which he would sip on as we chatted and talked.

He treated the small plastic bottle like someone would treat a whiskey flask—tucking it into his shirt or trouser pocket when not in use and revealing it on a whim, whenever the urge struck him. I tried to talk him into drinking cabanga instead of nipa, but he never did. Often he told me, "*Seu Cristiano . . . cabanga não dá* [doesn't get me drunk]; I need *nipa*." Whenever he visited my house, he would search through it looking for alcohol, and drink whatever he found. One time, this included a fifth of a bottle of imported whiskey. Not only did every-one in Caridade know of Antonio's dependence on alcohol, but the rest of the NGO and AIDS world in Pemba did as well. In spite of Antonio's occasionally poignant observations and criticisms of the government and medical establish-ment during district-level meetings, his behavior in other contexts infamously indicted Caridade as ineffective or not to be taken seriously. Within Caridade, we all wondered how it was possible that Antonio still held his official position as nurse, given his poor and unpredictable attendance at work. Remember that Antonio was also an ART patient and by this point had been on medication for several years.

Falume, Caridade's president of the assembly, had this to say about Antonio's drinking behavior:

Tem bom organismo, o gajo [the motherfucker has a strong body]! Very healthy! Without that, he couldn't keep up this *vicio* [vice]. He hardly eats, drinks *nipa* all the time, and rarely gets sick [with viral symptoms]. He is also smart, a very good nurse. He could be treating people in his own home if he wanted to. Instead, the only time you can catch him sober is if you get to his house as soon as he wakes up. Otherwise, it doesn't matter what he does or doesn't plan on doing that day. If he starts out for work, all it takes is one stop somewhere, anywhere, for a drink. From that point on, he won't show up at work, he just goes from drinking spot to drinking spot. When he starts this, you can see it happen, as if he changes into someone else. He takes the entire bottle of *nipa* in one gulp [Falume swallows harshly.], then the eyes get bloodshot and droop a little bit. Then, his body goes rigid [Falume locks his arms down at his side.] and finally loosens up [Falume slumps on his stool.]. At that point, he starts talking nonsense, and you know that he's gone. (Falume, AIDS association leader)

This, of course, explained Antonio's lack of interest in Caridade's regular activities and his excessive interest in paychecks.

On days when salaries were given out, if Antonio couldn't show up, he had another member walk the sum of money down to his home in Chipapwale. When he did appear to collect money, he usually didn't make it back home until the next morning. The drinking would begin immediately, first with a celebratory 2M beer, followed by barraca-bought gin, and finally his favorite substance, *nipa*. Carlitos would bring a reed mat outside for him to pass out on before he closed the office. One time, some Caridade activists were taking pictures of a passed-out Antonio on that mat after he had soiled himself, lying in dirty clothes, directly in the sunlight, in the middle of the day next to the office wall. Antonio's drinking affected the whole association, causing him to make bad decisions. We couldn't convince him to step down for the good of others. He hung on to his position as president, refusing to be ousted by other members and reacted violently to such suggestions. Likely, he wanted to continue funding his drinking habit and appreciated the prestige.

The power that he lauded over other members and activists, as a nurse in the day hospital and as president, demotivated and discouraged others from participation or from believing that the association would ever improve. When sober, he would make promises to people or commit to decisions that he couldn't keep, or would later overturn when he got drunk. The professionalism and behavior of other Caridade members were negatively impacted by all this. It wasn't that members emulated his behavior—nobody's drinking problem was as severe or frequent as Antonio's—but people took advantage of the chaos resulting from his poor and lackluster leadership. Before losing so much control over the association, Antonio also managed to install a few of his drinking friends (also

HIV-positive) into certain activist positions throughout the province, including in his home village of Mecufi. This further sullied the name of Caridade, perceived as a group of alcoholics who rarely did their job with precision. It made no sense, for example, to many local school teachers, why Caridade activists oversaw UNICEF school programs and were permitted to deliver HIV education to children.

Rita, also an HIV-positive Caridade activist dependent on *nipa*, owned a house in Chipapwale. She refused to sleep there because of threats from an ex-boyfriend. Instead, she spent her evenings in the homes of other boyfriends throughout the city. The NGO Medicos del Mundo, perhaps unaware of Rita's proclivity toward drinking, had installed her as an activist working in the bars and brothels of Pemba City. This position kept her both fed and opportunistically intoxicated, as she was offered meals or drinks from bar owners involved with the program. Others in Caridade suspected that Rita sometimes traded her own body for money or other goods when she was off duty. My own interactions with Rita became full of tension, as she invited herself to my home one day under the pretense of an interview.

After insisting that I buy beers and Cokes for us to drink, she suggested that we sleep together and that she become my girlfriend during the rest of my time in Pemba. When I refused, she spread rumors that this act had taken place anyway. Constantly tied up in court battles with ex-boyfriends, who she claimed would not return items left at their homes—items like radios, speakers, and clothing—Rita's social and economic situation deteriorated quickly. Medicos del Mundo found her drunk at an event for prevention education in a community police station, ending her activist salary and position. Her home in Chipapwale was flooded and broken into, leaving her truly destitute. As she refused to stop drinking, she blamed her problems on other people in Caridade—some of the same people who could have sheltered her during her continuing personal disasters.

Numerous other events raised concerns around the misuse of alcohol among activists in Pemba. When visitors from other associations came to the area—presidents and vice-presidents from other associations in other provinces, high-level activists in RENSIDA or from Maputo—they were courted and serenaded by Pemba-based activists who introduced them to the city's nightlife. Falume, the president of the assembly, was usually put in charge of identifying what bars to go to at what time, and what women might be suitable for the men, the *chefes* (bosses) on overnight trips to the area. I accompanied him on some of these outings and on multiple occasions, witnessed Maputo-based activists take home women from Pemba's bars.

For Caridade, on paydays, it was not unusual to find activists spending a good deal of their paycheck on drinks in the local *barracas*. Young females, somehow aware that it was payday, would show up to drink beer with association members, later disappearing with them into the alleyways as night fell. Some of the male activists also frequented brothels in Pemba City. There are many of these establishments, masquerading as hotels. Inside are rooms with at least two doors so that people can enter one side and leave through another. When I visited the homes of female activists, they would ask me to buy beer for them and would drink as many as I chose to provide to them. Luisa, Caridade's vice-president, was often found in the yard of her home drinking hard liquor. These behaviors were not anomalies; instead, they represented what was in Pemba a culture of drinking, sex, and escapism.

This aspect of local culture—alcoholism and partying—is an enormous challenge to treatment activism because it is so entrenched, accepted, and impactful. Clinicians certainly recognize the problem, linking the overconsumption of alcohol with a greater burden of HIV-related symptoms, low levels of social support, and new forms of stigma. The increasing emphasis on the nexus between treatment and alcohol, in mainstream published literature and in clinical studies, strongly suggests that this is yet another issue that cannot be comprehensively addressed in the clinic. It suggests the need for effective approaches to addiction at the community level—such as Alcoholics Anonymous (Valverde and White-Mair 1999), options that are free, publicly available, and operate independently—to be more accessible in this context. It also suggests the need for strategizing how the support group could be more involved with discouraging and limiting alcohol consumption among its members.

Of all the "subuniverses" where AIDS activism coexists, and must compete to establish itself and maintain legitimacy, the world of heavy drinking comprises a "marginal situation"—following Berger and Luckmann (1967: 97)—a "night side" of human life "that keeps lurking ominously on the periphery of everyday consciousness." The problems mentioned here are not anathema, although they take an effort to notice by getting out into the communities. The threat of alcoholism is prevalent in the lives of many ART patients in Pemba City, a place not all that unique in southern Africa. The idea that we cannot "treat" our way out of the HIV epidemic is underscored by realities such as these—that support for and among HIV-positive persons entails addressing sensitive life issues intertwined with compliance, domestic stability, and long-term possibilities for recovery.

For *ordinary people* living with HIV, substance abuse is a "syndemic" (Singer et al. 2017), an additional pathway for disease, and one that worsens its burden. Taking into account social and environmental factors—and ways toward recovery—could lead to effective amelioration. Further examining how and why AIDS activism could better address the scourge of alcohol abuse—and its associated behaviors, such as sexual promiscuity and domestic violence—begs greater research and attention now and in the future.

STILL MISSING: PRACTICAL
ACTIVISM FOR ORDINARY PEOPLE

The stories, statements, and encounters highlighted in this chapter expose topics of concern that are not well studied in the AIDS world—lingering confusion about the virus and the natures of activism, ineffective home-based care programs, rampant treatment abandonment, and alcoholism in Cabo Delgado Province. These have immense consequences for patients and implications for the future trajectory of activism as it unfolds in southern Africa. The intricacies and details of what goes on in Pemba and Cabo Delgado—what I suggest is a microcosm, a "subuniverse" of the wider struggle that patient-activists undergo and face—are not unique or isolated.

Likely, similar events are unfolding elsewhere and not receiving much scholarly attention or other publicity. The features of this subuniverse reveal that the provision of treatment, as well as the work of activists, is dysfunctional on several levels. HIV-positive persons are not obedient to biomedicine. They do not place much weight on the public work of activists. Their efforts and those of the state are viewed with ambiguity and not always trusted. Patients and activists—although they will use their HIV-positive status as leverage for resources—do not seek to stand out but rather want normality in life, stability in their domestic and social situations, and to be able to carry on with work and other personal endeavors. When treatment fits into this equation, it is embraced, not perfectly or consistently, but predictably and reliably for those who "know" that it is effective. There is some degree of treatment "activism" in anybody who fits this description.

Scholars of treatment activism emphasize its relevance as a human rights struggle and its capacity to transform people from subject to citizen, from a passive recipient to an active participant (Fenio 2011). This narrative takes on an air of civil rights and, unfortunately, of sociocultural evolution as well. Activists in Pemba are expected to conform to a better model, one that emphasizes outspokenness and the right to be demanding. Academics point to well-known success stories, like South Africa's TAC, which expanded and thrived on partnerships and the building of international and academic coalitions (Grebe 2011). In this way, HIV treatment activism gained widespread recognition and legitimacy as a politically oriented social movement, equipped to be, purportedly, active and present in virtually any setting. It successfully drew upon global agreements and worldwide treaties capable of empowering patients anywhere to make demands on the state and the culture around them, to be, in a word, "transformative activists" (Susser 2009: 142).

What happens, however, when chronicling the pursuits and lifestyles of HIV-positive persons in places like Pemba City is that this narrative either doesn't fit or begins to break down. The "common" activists described here do not have very clear understandings of human rights. Some default on their treatment. Others haven't even taken an HIV test. Groups carry out income-generating projects with a tendency to fail or that end up serving narrow interests. Unless they occupy a lower rung on an imaginary ladder of success—not yet modern or up to speed—then these activists are not given a clear category to occupy in the world of activism. They are, perhaps, "struggling," "imperfect," or "handicapped" activists whose positive intentions—and, indeed, a myriad of valid attempts and "little" achievements—nevertheless christen them as legitimate.

The subuniverse of Cabo Delgado Province does not flawlessly serve the oft-embraced agenda or stereotypes we have come to associate with treatment activism—that "some in Mozambique are becoming transnational citizens like their counterparts in South Africa" (Fenio 2011: 731) or that "those living with HIV/AIDS remake themselves as both citizens and humans, asserting 'who' they are through meaningful appearance in the public realm" (Hayden 2012: 587). Such assessments and statements do not apply to everyone and every place. It is possible that if and when they fail to fulfill particular criteria, subuniverses like the one in Cabo Delgado get "selected out," omitted, even dismissed as nonrepresentative or unimportant outliers. Unable to contribute to standard talking points, it is easier left unmentioned. Subuniverses, "like all social edifices of meaning," write Berger and Luckmann (1967: 84), "must be 'carried' by a particular collectivity."

It only follows that in a world of biosocial collectivities and biological citizens, some subuniverses are more privileged than others. If they resonate in the right way and at the right time, they can be taken for granted, permitted or nourished to represent and to speak on behalf of all the rest. Very successful and renowned activist groups come to be considered the establishment in the world of AIDS activism and to be taken as its "stable symbolic canopy" (Berger and Luckmann 1967: 86). Limited almost exclusively to treatment expansion, and having already done their job relatively well, these models may have little to offer moving forward.

The "triumph" of HIV treatment activism—getting ART into more and more public health facilities in southern Africa—is also, in some ways, the "triumph" of those who would like to see it end there, who can now claim "mission accomplished" and divert resources or attention to different emergencies, crises, or other deficiencies in international governance and development. The absorption of political resistance, the adoption of treatment into mainstream mechanisms of health care may—much like other attempts to make civil society voices heard and recognized (Tusalem 2007)—disproportionately favor the needs of the upper middle class over the lower. The evidence for this includes the longevity and persistence of very basic problems and challenges such as those elaborated upon in this chapter. Even with ready access to ARVs in clinics, patient-activists in Cabo Delgado still lack strong support groups and social networks. Average patients could very much benefit by having a greater say in the way the government manages AIDS associations and in the manner in which they are incorporated (or not) into the projects of NGOs.

Still missing are the practicalities of how to live well with HIV in Pemba City and in Cabo Delgado Province. Still missing are examples and models for a free and independent civil society. Still missing are sustained social relationships in a happy and thriving support group setting. Still missing are manifestations of a capable therapeutic community tailored to meet the needs of *ordinary people* so that they can overcome the right obstacles in this environment, where information is skewed and knowledge is too much subject to rumors and miscalculations. The needs and views of *ordinary people* are easily silenced and subsumed simply by placing—or claiming to place—drugs on the shelves of the clinic. Becoming more political—protests, demands, the elucidation of "rights" claims—as this next chapter will demonstrate, is not a valid strategy for everyone in all contexts. AIDS activism, in order to be successful, requires acknowledgment of its diversity and limitations and the development of various alternate forms and framings, even if they appear a bit different than what is considered to be the status quo.

5 · THE (DIS)INTEGRATION OF THE DAY HOSPITALS

On the morning of September 11, 2009, about a hundred AIDS activists gathered together in Pemba's *Praça dos Herois* (Hero Square), two kilometers away from the Provincial Health Office. Some had flown in from Maputo and others were trucked in from surrounding towns and villages, but most were association members and patients who had once attended Pemba's day hospital (*hospital de dia*, or HDD), the HIV treatment clinic that had closed down or, as the government phrased it, had been "integrated" into the main hospital. Participants planned to march along the city's main street, *Avenida 25 de Setembro*, with a letter to be hand delivered to the provincial health director, alerting him of their grievances. T-shirts with the slogan *HIV Positivo* were distributed to the participants, young people and adults alike, who had also prepared signs with phrases such as "Don't leave us to die!" "We are all equal," "You and I depend on treatment," and "No to stigma!" The biggest banner, the centerpiece in front of the marching crowd, contained the principal theme of the march. It read, "March for Life without Stigma—Pemba" Another one, almost as big, read, "Stop Stigma and Discrimination."

As people got into position, clustered with their organizations and friends, sirens from the police motorcycles guarding the protesters began to wail. A man with a megaphone—one of the Maputo-based activists—gave a quick speech: "We are all here as equals, and we know that what is happening in our country is wrong. People are suffering! Our brothers and sisters do not have the medical care they need! So what are we going to do about it? We are going to tell them what we think! And what do we think? Down with stigma!"

At this, the crowd responded, in unison, "Down with stigma!" and began marching forward. As the people progressed through the city's main thoroughfare, the administrative and commercial districts, microphones were brandished and the group chanted calls and responses. "We are all equal; we want better health; don't leave us to die!" People broke into song and danced happily in the caravan. Activists with their own motorcycles (including me) stayed in front, adding to the noise, and buzzing ahead a hundred meters or so whenever the crowd caught up with us. Just prior to ascending the final hill to the Provincial Health Office, one song in particular caught everyone's ear, adding much to the level of excitement. It was directed to the nation's minister of health, the enemy or villain of this activist campaign. The group sang, "Ivo Garrido, you have really done it this time!"

Stationing themselves on the manicured lawn outside the main entrance to the provincial health director's office, people continued to shout phrases like "Better health care!" and "We want more centers!" Some journalists in the crowd started conducting interviews for radio and television. "We need to see doctors! Down with stigma! We are not dried fish! Where is Doctor Cesário? Where is Nurse Inês? Where is the food we have been promised? We want better nutrition!" It was extremely hot and despite continued attempts to keep the energy high—some impromptu speeches, additional singing, brief improvisational comedy sketches of the minister of health closing down HIV clinics—the crowd began to dwindle. After two hours of waiting, the director had still not appeared, and people were leaving to seek shade, water, and food. A group of office workers started to gather outside, telling the group to leave the premises.

Grabbing a megaphone, Luisa—Caridade's vice-president, who had been appointed leader of the protests—directed her voice toward the building with the intention of being clearly heard. She stated that these same protests were going on right now in other cities. In Lichinga, Quelimane, Xai-Xai, and Tete, activists were marching and gathering this same day and for the same exact cause. "If the director is not going to come outside, I will read the letter to him myself!" she stated. At that, and with the letter in her hand, she motioned for two other activists to accompany her, and they marched toward the entrance to the building. They were forcefully stopped by armed guards and retreated back onto the lawn where most of us were still standing.

We got word that some activists had spotted the provincial health director attempting to leave in a Ministry of Health vehicle, but they had blocked the entrance to the parking lot with their bodies, forcing him to go back inside. A few minutes later, he finally emerged, dressed in a suit and tie and sweating profusely. Luisa approached him with the letter in hand, but he barely made eye contact with her and addressed the rest of the crowd instead. "What do you have to say to me, personally?" he asked. "I don't have time for these *brincadeiras* [games]!" Luisa waved the letter in his face tauntingly. Fuming, he snatched the letter from her hand and said he would read it inside, at his desk, but not here in public.

After this, the protest ended, very disappointingly. Some people trickled out of the crowd and back to their homes. Others returned to the staging area, waiting for the trip back out to their village or town. The Pemba Provincial Health Office never issued a response, but Mozambican news and media took notice. There were headlines in local newspapers and online (IRIN PlusNews 2009b). However, nothing really came from the effort. The HDDs never reopened, and no other show of force was made on behalf of HIV-positive patients in Pemba. This was the first HIV treatment protest in Pemba, making the results more discouraging of similar, future endeavors.

The Pemba protest was in a sense contrived, coordinated by a small group of activists based in Maputo who dubbed themselves the *Liga contra Discriminação* (Antidiscrimination League). The motivations for the protest, however, were quite authentic not only in Pemba but in the rest of the nation as well. People with HIV were upset at the integration—or really, the disintegration—of their treatment centers, the HDDs that had been the locus of HIV treatment distribution since its early stages in the country. Yet the letter that Luisa handed to the provincial health director, a carbon copy of the one handed to the minister of health in Maputo during a similar protest a month earlier, made no mention of HDDs or the closures. Demands to reopen the facilities had been removed and replaced with vague ones, requests for better services and less stigma, because the activists had been forewarned—by their own government—that the clinics were gone forever.

The reason for this was because HIV treatment, according to the state, should not be limited to HDDs alone but "decentralized" to all health units. Ivo Garrido, the minister of health, noted that HIV-positive patients should not be forced to congregate in one place and even went so far as to label day hospitals a "foci of discrimination" (Olsen 2013: 243). This was an assessment quite opposite to that of the patients themselves, who appreciated the convenience and discretion afforded them by having their own facilities. Faced with the state's claim that more patients could be reached by devolving services into the national health system, activists in Mozambique, despite a preference for having their own HIV/AIDS clinics, were robbed of their traditional mantra—that people with HIV are the same as everybody else and that treatment should be provided for free everywhere. The state, apparently, had taken activists up on their request of providing universal health care but in a way that did not seem to privilege them.

In this chapter, I suggest that the broadly resonant "master frame" (Porta and Diani 2006; Benford and Snow 2000) of politically oriented HIV treatment activism—more treatment, for more people, in more places—has failed and even done a disservice to patient-activists in Mozambique. Enormous and disproportionate attention has been paid to HIV/AIDS patients and their protests or rights claims, resulting in a preference for a mode of interpretation establishing injustice and victimization as the justification for their existence. What occurs when this justification is taken away from them is the perceived subsequent irrelevance of the movement itself.

Since the inception of the "movement," HIV-positive activists have been portrayed as primarily interested in treatment access (Smith and Siplon 2006). The wider struggle for social justice, and even for complete unity among the movement's adherents, is seen as insurmountable compared to just getting a prescription for a drug or a pill. In the second decade of the 2000s, however, this overarching mobilizing structure (Tarrow and Tilly 2009)—of poor treatment access and perceived stigma and discrimination—has become impermanent, absorbed, and is beginning to be addressed by the very same entities and powers that were previously considered the movement's targeted enemies. A poor selection of case studies—a focus on ACT UP or TAC and similar groups engaged in open dissent—has lent itself well to imprecision and biases that hindered the further testing and refinement of additional proposals about what treatment activism is, does, and could be in other real-world settings.

Early scholarship on HIV treatment activism was dominated by what some scholars call "political process theorists" (Jasper 2014), who view the study of protests, social disruption, and rights-based challenges to political oppression as their end goal. This leads to stagnation and a focus more on the emergence of a social movement than the viability of its form, strategies, or impacts. Political process theorists remain enamored of overarching, supposedly universal models used by some social movements to challenge power. Latching on to the political opportunity thesis, the main argument of this approach is that people join social movements primarily as a response to political opportunities and then, working together, seek to open up new ones (Tarrow 2011).

The inherent implication is that political involvement is sufficient for social movement mobilization. It also presumes a fight, a consistent back and forth between those with and without power. For political process theorists, social movements are "collective challenges by people with common purposes and solidarity in sustained interaction with elites, opponents, and authorities" (Tarrow 2011: 3–4). If these elites, opponents, or authorities manage to remove themselves from the fray—by, for example, agreeing on some points with activists themselves—then the movement has nothing against which to struggle and is likely to fall flat.

In this chapter, I will explain how this occurred in the context of the "decentralization" of Mozambican day hospitals. As part of a wider international trend toward "health systems strengthening" (Abt Associates Inc. 2012; WHO 2007), the traditional "master frame" of AIDS activism—treatment equity, maximizing the number of beneficiaries of ART—was relocated from the street into institutions and transformed from being radical to mainstream. Health systems strengthening is an example of what happens when the "policy implementation capacity" (Rucht 2007: 254) of the state is too broad and not subject to local-level, democratic discussion or debate. It essentially robbed activists of their elite allies, who could now support treatment expansion via ways and means less outside of their comfort zone.

This unfolding of events suggests that describing protest should not be the aim of research, at least not without filling in more of the blanks. Protests are easily, and usually, sensationalized. Treatment activists, defined principally by political process theory, found themselves unable to shape what occurred around them and unable to adapt to the shifting constellations of change happening around their own health care. In that particular iteration, AIDS activism, dominated by concerns mostly for biomedical therapy and by activists interested in airing their grievances more in public than in private, was destined for decline and obsolescence.

DAY HOSPITAL CLOSURES

The HDD closures should not have come as a surprise to AIDS activists. It was being discussed at least two years before it occurred. During my first trip to Mozambique, in 2007, the topic came up repeatedly in interviews with activists in Maputo and Pemba. When queried on their opinions, however, the responses were strikingly ambiguous. Patients then were much more open to the idea of a day hospital integration: "The hospitals are full, and the day hospitals are few. They should integrate them because the central hospitals don't have what they need. Also, people really do abandon their treatment because of the day hospital. Nobody wants to be seen there. We are all people, we are all patients, and diseases are diseases. So it is a good idea to join the hospitals together" (Alfonso, MATRAM activist).

There was an acknowledgment that resources were not evenly distributed and that getting rid of day hospitals might be the solution: "There is this big access problem in the rural areas and no trained health care personnel. So I see what they are trying to do. Patients should not have to come to the cities just to get treatment, and when they try to get ARVs in a rural area and are not well received, they might not come back again. So there has to be some equality there" (João, MATRAM activist).

On the point of discrimination, some patients emphasized the desire for confidentiality over simply having their own clinic facility and the ultimate need to protect their positive status from involuntary disclosure to others: "People pass by the day hospital and make nasty comments. They're just not very nice! So yes, some people are scared to come to the day hospital for fear they will be spotted there. But in the main hospital, it's obvious to anyone who sees my [health] card that I'm HIV positive. So it's hard to tell where the discrimination might be worse, here or there" (Aleny, MATRAM activist).

Yet patients were also keenly aware that they would lose something along with their day hospitals, in particular, convenience and some degree of specialty care:

> Treatment for someone who is seropositive is different than from a normal patient. And if they integrate, the waiting time for us in the hospitals would be intolerable! Now I go to the day hospital in the morning and am finished by 1 p.m. If they integrate, I would have to come back the next day [for a test or laboratory result]. (Samwel, MATRAM activist)

> The doctors in the day hospital know what they are doing and work very well, so integrating them is a bad idea because there the doctors treat HIV only. I have never heard of a drug shortage in a day hospital, but our other hospitals don't function. If they integrate, there will be nothing there for us [HIV patients]. Those other hospitals don't have health technicians or laboratories; stigma is worse there. If this happens, where will we get our medications? (Antonio, MATRAM activist)

While many people were very aware that "an integration" was being considered, they did not know when or how it might actually happen. The order was given to close the HDDs in early 2008, and, at least initially, Ivo Garrido denied it was even true. This was a source of much angst and fear among ART patients. The newspaper report—perhaps on the basis of an inadvertent leak by the Ministry of Health, according to discussions I had with health care staff—indicated that discussion between patients and the government on this topic probably should have ensued much earlier:

> Mozambican Health Minister Ivo Garrido has denied that he ever ordered the closure of the "Day Hospitals" which cater solely for HIV-positive patients, according to a report in Friday's issue of the independent weekly "Savana." It has taken the Minister a month to deny the story, which first appeared in the 27 February issue of the Maputo daily "Noticias." The paper claimed that Garrido decided to close the Day Hospitals because he regarded such separate treatment as contributing to the stigmatization of, and discrimination against people suffering from HIV/AIDS. "The Day Hospitals have no place in the structure of the Ministry of Health," said Garrido, as cited by "Noticias." Regardless of the beliefs of those who had set them up, they had become foci of discrimination against AIDS patients "and that's why I have decided to abolish

them." No letter from the Health Ministry denying this story appeared, and "Noticias" never published any retraction. Furthermore the closure of the Day Hospitals seemed to be in line with Ministry policy. According to "Savana," NGOS that work on HIV/AIDS say that the decision to integrate anti-retroviral treatment for HIV-positive people into the normal services of the health units, rather than keeping it as something separate, was taken over a year ago. Nonetheless, the "Noticias" story created some alarm among the patients who were using the Day Hospitals, who had not been prepared for any change in their method of treatment. Some told reporters they feared for their survival if they had to receive treatment from units not specialised in HIV/AIDS matters. Such concerns may have led to a quiet volte-face. For speaking to reporters last Tuesday, during an interval in a meeting of the Health Ministry's Coordinating Council, Garrido declared that he had not ordered the closure of the Day Hospitals, and that they are still functioning. He added that all measures taken by the Health Ministry "seek to guarantee the well-being of patients and not to damage their interests." (Savana 2008)

Nevertheless, over the course of the next year, day hospitals began closing, slowly but surely. One by one they were "integrated" into the main hospital, often with no warning or notice given to patients about what was to occur (IRIN Plus-News 2009a). When this began, some patients knew about it, and others found out the hard way. Activists—who, perhaps, should have been aware—were too slow to address what appears to have been a systematic removal of HDDs until much too late. Nobody, including the health workers and day hospital staff themselves, was really prepared.

The way this "integration" happened differed from site to site. In some cities, like Chimoio, the day hospital doors were locked and patients were redirected to the central hospital waiting area. In other places, like some sites in Maputo, patients were told to report to other wings—a "Department for Chronic Disease" (Olsen 2013: 231). These tended to be dilapidated buildings with a new name but still devoted mostly to HIV-positive patients—the most common type of chronically ill person. They often found themselves waiting outside in the sun and even more exposed to the eyes of passersby than they had been in their original sites. One of the official reasons given for "integrating" the day hospitals was to bring treatment closer to the homes of patients.

Olsen (2013) notes that attempts to do this failed. In many cases, patients did not want to be seen obtaining treatment close to their homes and went to other neighborhoods, sometimes traveling great distances to do so. Some clinics became congested and others became empty because patients did not show up where they were always expected to. Now, for the first time since HIV treatment began in Mozambique, ARV drug shortages became a widespread concern. After the day hospital "integration," providers began only partially filling prescriptions—giving half a month's number of pills or less—requesting patients to come back frequently to check and see when more pills were available (PBS Newshour 2010).

In Pemba, one of the last sites to be "integrated," the day hospital building remained in use but was transformed into an auxiliary waiting and triage area for the central hospital. HIV-positive patients arriving there were surprised to find it overflowing with strangers and people suffering from a variety of other ailments from broken arms to tuberculosis to malaria. HIV-related work was supposed to continue as normal, but it didn't. Activists who worked with new patients to carry out treatment counseling, for example, had no space in which to do it. Education on HIV, normally carried out with a TV/VCR or a flipchart of illustrations in the corner of the waiting area, ceased because there was barely any room for a teacher to stand. Noise levels were too high to speak over.

Also, the day hospital staff had been split up. Some were transferred to other wings of the hospital, others to entirely different clinics in the city. Patients, who previously knew staff by name, were now faced with new health care workers not only unfamiliar with their specific cases but also not well trained (if at all) in the area of HIV. Inside the former day hospital, doorways had pieces of paper taped to the front as signs with the words "pediatrics," "maternity," or "triage" on them. There was no longer a consulting room only for HIV patients. Laboratory equipment had been consolidated into one room, and the workers were cramped inside. The HIV testing center, next door, was also shut down. It had been taken over as offices for the Elizabeth Glazer Pediatric AIDS Foundation, a PEPFAR contractor.

Patients had mixed reactions to the loss of the day hospital. Some were in favor of it: "I appreciate the joining of the two hospitals. The changes are good because everyone used to say that this hospital had AIDS. Now it is better, it eliminates discrimination. In the past, everyone knew that the day hospital was special. Now everyone is together, so I prefer it this way" (Marcos, ART patient).

The day hospital did embarrass some patients, who believed that it was easier for them to hide their status from others according to the new arrangements and were perfectly happy to not be seen in an HIV/AIDS clinic:

Hospitals were not originally integrated into African societies at all! Now, again, we are rid of these outside influences [he refers to the NGOs who ran the day hospital]. People still go in, just look at all of the doorways, they can hide in those rooms and nobody knows the difference. Now that there is no separation, there is less discrimination, so it is a good thing. The government knows what they are doing. Now you can't tell the difference between patients. There is less suspicion. It was so strange before. (Alex, ART patient)

It is better now. In order to do anything else in the hospital, people have to get a test first [she mistakenly believed an HIV test was now required for anyone at all to be seen in the hospital]. Now we will know everyone who has the virus, so this is good for the community. The change is normal, I can still hide my medication. My children ask me every day, "Mom, you are taking pills?" but they do not know what the pills are. (Felicitas, ART patient)

Not all agreed, however, and various people spoke up against the day hospital "integration":

It was better to have our own hospital. Everyone is looking at us, they won't eat with us. People have stopped coming for their ARVs. This is a complex disease, it needs to be controlled. This way, there is less control [referring to laboratory tests and patient assessments]. (Azimo, ART patient)

Many people with HIV already are not registered [for ART]. They usually arrive too late for treatment anyway. How can this be better for them, who were scared to come even then [before the integration]? If you look around, nobody even does lectures anymore [HIV/AIDS education] because they don't get paid. I will still come here, there isn't another option, but I do not think that the government is hearing what we patients are saying. (Marcia, ART patient)

At first this was a discriminatory place, the "door of AIDS," people called it. Now it is gone, but for what? Now look, the space is gone, there are no beds, there are longer waiting periods. And the others here now are talking bad about us, saying, "Why did they put us here with HIV patients?" In the pharmacy too, when you hand over your card, you can start to feel ashamed and people talk about it. It was better *entre nos* [between us only]. (Peter, ART patient)

Experiences with the "integration" were highly varied, which suggests that the process was not standardized. There were, most likely, severe deficiencies in its implementation. In Pemba, for example, the integration was unarguably messy. Attempts were not made to clarify how it would happen, what new roles activists would undertake, or to introduce new staff to them. Activists were questioned about their legitimacy in the new hospital spaces and found it difficult to do their jobs:

I arrived one day to begin my normal duties when a health technician I don't know asked me what I was doing here. I replied, "*Senhor*, I am an activist, and I am here to work with the HIV patients." One patient waiting for a consultation told me to leave, that we don't need dirty people in the hospital. As I argued with that man, the health worker told me to be quiet, to stop making noise. I didn't go home, I stayed to do my job, but felt ashamed and demoralized. Who are these new people, and why don't they like us? Why are they trying to make us feel isolated and keep us from doing our jobs? (Albertina, AIDS activist)

There was also misunderstanding about how far reaching the process had been. Some were unaware that day hospitals were closed down nationally and blamed it on local authorities:

That Dr. Saúde [the former day hospital health technician] is not doing a good job. Why did he close the pharmacy in the day hospital? And without telling us he was going to do it? [I explain to him it was a national decision, not one made in Pemba by Dr. Saúde.] OK, but the least they could have done was explain to the patients what was happening. None of us understand what is happening in the hospital. (Ricard, home-based care patient)

Some effort could have been made to communicate what was happening so that patients had fewer questions and knew what to expect. This, however, may not have been a priority for the government.

As discussed in chapter 2, the issue of HDDs in Mozambique has always been relatively unstable and somewhat tense. Kalofonos (2008) noted that, in 2004, they were introduced to offset stigma—that HIV-positive people did not feel safe in standard hospital environments—but also for surveillance purposes and to control medication stock. HIV was then still very much considered an emergency, and the country welcomed outside help. ARVs were expensive and so donors insisted on a direct route to patients that was free from government bureaucracy and inefficiency. The Ministry of Health was at first on board with the idea. HDDs, when first starting up, were not supposed to be set apart from the rest of the health system. They were initially labeled as "specialty units *integrated* into the existing network of health services . . . places for the introduction and control of anti-retroviral therapy" (MISAU 2004: 7; my emphasis). However, their implementation occurred at a time of increased donor interest in HIV/AIDS that may have seemed threatening to national sovereignty.[1] Therefore, the Ministry of Health may have always harbored some mistrust and skepticism about a system not entirely under its control (see chapter 2).

Over time, through NGO support and a disproportionate amount of international funding, many day hospitals became relatively independent. Some—especially those built and run by international medical NGOs—had more reliable services than government hospitals, better equipment, and higher staff-to-patient ratios. HDDs were insulated spaces. HIV-positive patients could be referred out—pregnant women, for example, or those in need of physical rehabilitation—but HIV-negative patients could never be referred in, making HDDs efficient but otherwise limited and noncollaborative. This sparked jealousy and contempt. Over time, day hospitals came under fire as NGO creations, poorly linked to other health services and incapable of contributing to the advancement of the nation's health system (Pfeiffer et al. 2010). Increasingly, it was argued that arrangements such as these—programs and specialty clinics targeting one disease only—were inequitable (Schneider et al. 2006).

According to this understanding, it was preferable, as much as possible, to minimize distances from home to clinic, maximize client usage and the number of beneficiaries, and introduce ARV services in as many sites as possible (Grépin 2011; Van Damme and Kegels 2006). These and similar arguments may have emboldened the Mozambican Ministry of Health to begin doing away with HDDs in the country—a system that had seen ART coverage rise from 3 percent in 2003 to either 13 or 56 percent in 2008, depending on how we stack the numbers[2] (MISAU 2015). Note that, in 2016, coverage was estimated at 65 percent of adult positives (MISAU 2017a).

Some within the activist community were more in tune with the broader, symbolic implications of these closures than other patients. Day hospitals had become, in a sense, political chess pieces in a fight between the ministry and humanitarian NGOs. César, the director of MATRAM in Maputo (the access-to-treatment movement), told me his opinion—that the Ministry of Health was so incompetent and so poorly structured that it could never get HIV treatment right. Foreign NGOs, many of which staffed and ran day hospitals, had to stay and continue with their projects, perpetually. The ministry was intimidated by this prospect and more interested in asserting their power and domination than with actually helping patients.

Likely, according to César, government policy would move in whatever direction necessary to kick NGOs out of HIV treatment—an intervention over which the government now wanted total credit for implementing. "Democracy kills," he told me. "Instead of improving things, the people in charge just want to show everybody that 'I am the boss.'" He lamented the language being used to describe what was in his mind a step backward and, potentially, a large-scale attack on civil society. The "integration" would concentrate more political power in Maputo and give politicians greater control over patient's lives. "When they do decentralize everything," he said, "it means people here [in Maputo] will have access to everything in the rest of the country."[3]

As I began to ask more questions about the day hospitals and their closures in organizations around Maputo, two main camps began to emerge—and some continued to throw this word, "decentralization," around in their dialogue. The first camp consisted of AIDS activists, such as César of MATRAM, and people in international NGOs working at the clinic level, who found the move disheartening. "We put a lot of time and money into these facilities," said the Doctors without Borders (MSF-Switzerland) education coordinator. "The patients do well there. It is their place." She alluded to an army of patient-activists operating with the support of groups like MSF. I asked her what the options were at this point. She responded, "The government is very clear that [the day hospitals] will close. There is nothing to be done about that. In their place, we are planning to open HIV/AIDS 'centers.' They won't have the same types of services—like medication and hospital care—but we can do some things. We are thinking along the lines of nutrition counseling, education, and employment services" (Lilith, international NGO worker).

The suggestion revealed the perceived benefits of day hospitals as much more than just treatment related. The desire to see these continue served as motivation enough for MSF to begin considering alternatives—HIV/AIDS "centers"—to counteract the rapid closing down of day hospitals, which was occurring without warning. An MSF doctor in the Tete day hospital said, "They just barged in one day, and we were told to leave by the next." Faced with, basically, a government-enforced shutdown, they had no time to notify patients, reorganize project staff, or close out basic activities. "It was sudden, and we were anything but prepared," he told me when I interviewed him in Washington, D.C., five years later.

The other camp consisted of program coordinators of multinational institutions, such as UNAIDS and the CDC. Their opinions about closing down the day hospitals were almost opposite that of the first camp. They embraced the understanding that ART, by any means, had to be provided in more clinic sites. In the name of equity and better distribution, day hospitals had to be eliminated. "The day hospitals are being collapsed as part of an overall project of decentralization," said the director of UNAIDS, Mauricio Cysne, in Maputo. "Just with the sheer numbers of people living with HIV here, the day hospitals could even get bigger than regular clinic facilities. It will be easier for the government to better track patients this way. HIV patients are just like everybody else. They suffer from the same diseases that other people all over the world suffer from, so they need to be able to access all of the other services in the hospital. The activists are another problem."

When I asked him about that last point, the UNAIDS director began to address the patient's fundamental right to privacy and to not be identified by any other party as HIV positive: "How would you feel if strangers could go into a hospital and look at your medical records? Such a thing would be unheard of in Michigan [where my university was located]. These AIDS associations and activists are not part of the U.N. system, so we are not particularly interested in working with them."

I mentioned to him that the activists, nonetheless, felt insulted, as if their efforts to help get people on treatment went unappreciated. They had frequent contact with other patients and believed that treatment program retention would suffer if the day hospitals were taken away. His response was that "this integration is going to happen. We don't know what this will look like on the ground, but the theory is sound." When told that AIDS activists were complaining about the day hospital closures, an expatriate CDC worker told me, "We need data. If they are going to complain about this, we need data because in other places what we are seeing is that putting money just into HIV doesn't help the rest of the country's patients."

Ivo Garrido—the man who, upon "decentralizing" the day hospitals, would soon be the prime target of AIDS activists' ire—fell firmly into this second camp of opinions. This camp was composed of experts and foreign-born workers in charge of large-scale programs who did not see eye-to-eye with the smaller, field-based humanitarian NGOs like MSF. It was, perhaps, mildly surprising that Garrido fell into any camp of opinions along with foreigners. A staunch Frelimo party nationalist, he is famous for enforcing certain parts of the "Kaya Kwanga Commitment" (WHO 2000), a framework issued by the Ministry of Health to regulate the perceived incursion of NGO interests within the nation's borders. His efforts to assign foreign health workers to isolated, rural areas of Mozambique were construed as particularly bold, even dictatorial, by NGOs that had no intention of opening offices or supporting staff in the places he determined were most in need. If by closing down the HDDs Garrido was carrying on with this type of a mission—controlling foreign interests and ensuring compliance with the needs of the nation—it is one that he never used as a defense. What he did say when finally confronted by AIDS activists in Maputo was similar to what the UNAIDS director and the CDC worker told me when I interviewed them almost five months prior.

Four to five hundred activists marched in the Maputo protest. Carrying signs, chanting, and wearing "HIV Positivo" T-shirts, they approached the Ministry of Health building where Dr. Garrido, aware of the effort, was waiting to greet them. He stood patiently by as César of MATRAM, on national television and radio, read aloud the letter calling him a "dictator" for closing the day hospitals and not consulting the patients. "We want to express our indignation over the process of these closures," said César. He mentioned specific cases where patients had been discriminated against, that wait times had increased, and that medication in some sites had become unavailable. New hospital staff, he said, did not have the "patience" to attend cases of HIV/AIDS as they did in the day hospitals (DREAM 2009).

Given a chance to respond, Garrido did so mostly in the affirmative. Of course, he said, all of these concerns would be taken into account. Of course, he said, patients would continue to receive the highest possible care that the country could provide. In fact, they had no need to worry because even more attention was going to be paid to them in the near future. But the topic of the day hospitals was not up for debate, they no longer had a part in the Mozambican HIV/AIDS planning process (Verdade 2009). The word that he used to describe the process was "decentralization." "If we had to open a day hospital at every place where HIV patients are being treated, we would end up with two national health systems. From a public health perspective, this is impossible," he told the crowd (Agência de Notícias de Resposta ao SIDA 2009). Garrido also claimed that the decision to "abolish" the day hospitals was his own, and it was irreversible. Over and over again, in the newspapers, on radio, and in television interviews, Ivo Garrido reasserted that the day hospital closures were his decision and that they were being "integrated" and "decentralized" into the main hospital system.

Over the course of the next two months, the rest of the day hospitals were shut down, including the one in Pemba.[4] Carrying out additional protests, as described at the beginning of this chapter, had no apparent impact on the ministry's actions. It was difficult to tell, in 2009, what effect closing the day hospitals had on patients. Activist groups, like MATRAM and its associates, estimated that 40 percent had at some point either dropped out or interrupted treatment as services changed (IRIN PlusNews 2009c). Some advocates might argue that decentralization was responsible for increased ART coverage in Mozambique. In 2016, 72 percent of primary clinics offered treatment (versus only 15 percent in 2009) and 64 percent of adults living with HIV were enrolled (MISAU 2017a).

But while these are laudable evolutions, they were slow to unfold, confirming the fears protesters had about the sudden shutdown of the HDDs. By 2012, three years after the closure of the HDDs, the number of clinics offering ART was just seven percentage points higher (at 22 percent), and the number of adults in treatment had risen just nine percentage points (also to 22 percent). While the biggest gains came between 2013 and 2015, most patients on ART—75 percent of them, according to UNAIDS (UNAIDS 2016)—are still treated in just 20 percent of health facilities and mostly in bigger cities like Maputo.

Rising HIV prevalence rates are another disappointment. While rates have gone modestly down in three provinces, from 2009 to 2015, prevalence has risen in all six others and Maputo City, in some cases alarmingly (see figure 5.1[5] and table 5.1;[6] INS 2015; INS 2010). Cabo Delgado is one such place, where prevalence rose by 46 percent overall (from 9.4 to 13.8). Though these provincial level changes don't affect the national numbers all that much—prevalence rose less than two percentage points (from 11.5 to 13.2) for the country overall—the problem is compounded within specific groups, generally the poor and more vulnerable.

Among those without any education, for example, prevalence increased between three and four percentage points regardless of gender (from 9.3 to

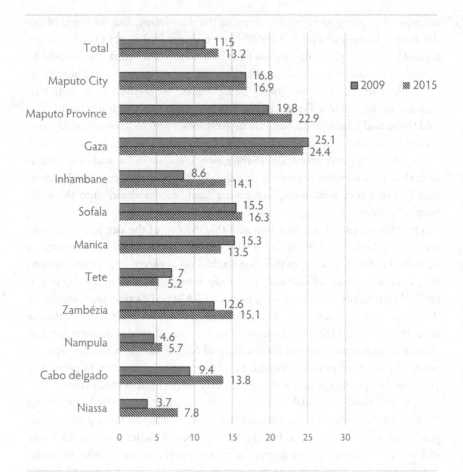

FIGURE 5.1. Percentages of women and men age fifteen to forty-nine years old who are HIV positive by province, Mozambique, 2009 and 2015

13.2 percent, again see table 5.1). The same is true for Mozambicans who earn the least money, with the starkest example being women in the lowest "wealth quintile" (from 6.6 to 10.4 percent). The only decreases at the national level are among urban men (one-half of one percentage point), men with secondary schooling, and Mozambicans at the highest wealth quintile regardless of gender.

Besides prevalence, there are other troubling outcomes around HIV/AIDS after decentralization. Knowledge of basic HIV prevention methods—use of condoms and having one uninfected partner—has decreased (figure 5.2).[7] Comprehensive knowledge about HIV—which includes condoms but also misconceptions like HIV spreading through mosquito bites—is also down, especially among adult men (figure 5.3)[8] and young men fifteen to twenty-four

TABLE 5.1   HIV prevalence by socioeconomic characteristics, 2009 to 2015

	Women		Men		Total	
	2009 (%)	2015 (%)	2009 (%)	2015 (%)	2009 (%)	2015 (%)
Residence						
Urban	18.4	20.5	12.8	12.3	15.9	16.8
Rural	10.7	12.6	7.2	8.6	9.2	11
Education level						
No education	9.8	13.8	7.2	10.8	9.3	13.2
Primary school	14.4	16.1	9.1	10.5	12.1	13.7
Secondary school	15	15.7	10.1	9.2	12.1	12.2
Wealth quintile						
Lowest	6.6	10.4	5	8.4	6	9.6
second	8.6	9.9	5.9	7.1	7.5	8.7
Middle	9.9	13.8	7.3	8.8	8.8	11.7
Fourth	18.3	21.1	12.6	14	16	18.3
Highest	20.6	20.4	13.5	11.3	17.4	16.2
Province						
Niassa	3.3	10.3	4.3	4.5	3.7	7.8
Cabo Delgado	9.5	15.7	9.2	11.4	9.4	13.8
Nampula	5.5	5.1	3.3	6.5	4.6	5.7
Zambézia	15.3	16.8	8.9	12.5	12.6	15.1
Tete	8	6.4	5.7	3.3	7	5.2
Manica	15.6	15.6	14.8	10.3	15.3	13.5
Sofala	17.8	18.8	12.6	13	15.5	16.3
Inhambane	10	17.7	5.8	7.6	8.6	14.1
Gaza	29.9	28.2	16.8	17.6	25.1	24.4
Maputo Province	20	29.6	19.5	15.8	19.8	22.9
Maputo City	20.5	21.7	12.3	11	16.8	16.9
Total	13.1	15.4	9.2	10.1	11.5	13.2

years old (figure 5.4).[9] Also, after a spike in 2011, knowledge of mother-to-child transmission prevention is falling (figure 5.5).[10] Glaring at statistics such as these, plotted as static or falling lines on troubling graphs, makes it seem like the health system "flattened out" instead of improved. While causality cannot simply be traced to the HDD closures, some changes that occurred around that time have had a clear negative impact.

Decentralization, while it has not delivered on its promise of putting ART on the shelves of every health unit or decreasing the burden of HIV in Mozambique, did accomplish one great feat. It reduced the presence and influence of

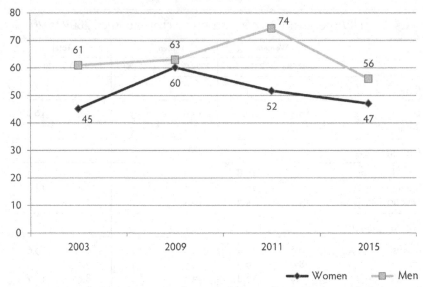

FIGURE 5.2. Percentages of women and men age fifteen to forty-nine years old who, in response to prompted questions, say that people can reduce the risk of getting HIV by using condoms every time they have sexual intercourse and by having one sex partner who is not infected and has no other partners, Mozambique, 2003 to 2015

humanitarian NGOs in favor not just of the state but of larger, more powerful and influential "global health initiatives" (GHIs, such as PEPFAR). As the HDDs got decentralized, coordinators in Cabo Delgado told me they now occupied only a "support role" in the health system. They were tasked with diversifying their programming to support other diseases and instructed not to focus on HIV/AIDS alone. MONASO, the government NGO in charge of administering to AIDS associations, also began to lose funding and relevance.

Thus while HDDs and the international NGOs that worked most closely with activists and patients faded into the background, other features of a targeted HIV/AIDS response in Mozambique continued to function unhindered, as long as they benefited the state and the government. The Núcleos and the National AIDS Council continued to operate, and their offices remained open. The Provincial Health Offices retained their strategic plans, HIV/AIDS specialty staff, and task force meetings. Select programs, such as ECOSida—an HIV project directed toward the private sector and business community—were more actively promoted after decentralization than before. The number of "community-based organizations," a term given to PEPFAR contractors, rapidly increased, and the scope of their involvement grew as they were planted in provincial capitals all over the country. UNAIDS was not slimmed down, but RENSIDA—the national network of people with AIDS

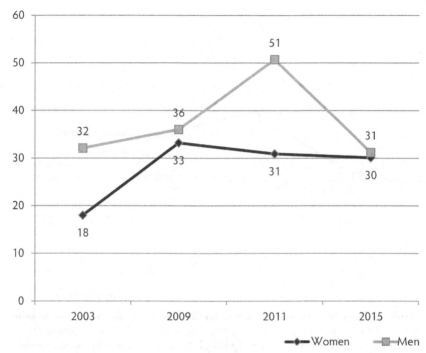

FIGURE 5.3. Percentages of women and men age fifteen to forty-nine years old who know that the consistent use of condoms during sexual intercourse and having just one uninfected partner can reduce the chances of getting HIV, know that a healthy-looking person can have HIV, and reject the two most common local misconceptions about transmission or prevention of HIV (that it can be contracted through mosquito bites or eating with an HIV-positive person), Mozambique, 2003 to 2015

and a U.N.-funded project—was significantly restructured and subject to massive staff changes and reductions.

The implementation of decentralization applied a double standard, one that favored the largest national and international entities over the smallest. The justification for decentralization—doing away with AIDS exceptionalism and the parallel health system of day hospitals—applied only to patient clinics and their friendly parties but not to well-funded bureaucratic structures, even if there was overlap between them. Given Mozambique's long-standing reliance on foreign HIV/AIDS strategies, Garrido's assertion that HDD closures were only his decision is questionable.

Mauricio Cysne, the UNAIDS director, was quoted at the time making very similar comments as Garrido. "The day hospitals can't be managed. We can't confirm that this is the model for putting 1.5 million people on treatment," reported IRIN PlusNews (2009c). The report continued, "Following Cysne, the decentralization idea permits the patient to receive services closer

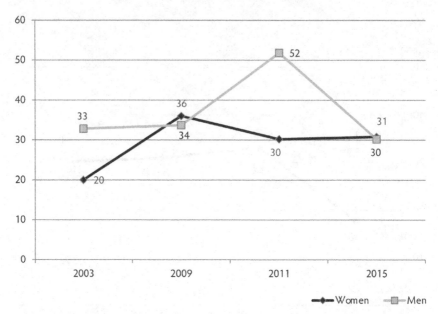

FIGURE 5.4. Percentages of women and men age fifteen to twenty-four years old who know that the consistent use of condoms during sexual intercourse and having just one uninfected partner can reduce the chances of getting HIV, know that a healthy-looking person can have HIV, and reject the two most common local misconceptions about transmission or prevention of HIV (that it can be contracted through mosquito bites or eating with an HIV-positive person), Mozambique, 2003 to 2015

to home. The day hospitals are too far away. . . . Decentralization would be, according to Cysne, the only way to transform into reality the guarantee that patients can access universal treatment and a basic health services package" (my translation).

While Ivo Garrido was certainly the "face" of the decentralization of day hospitals, his decision to close these hospitals did not occur in an information vacuum. Others, at top levels of the nation's development industry, shared his opinion. About a year later, Ivo Garrido was sacked from his position, and the new health minister continued to struggle with the impacts of the HDD closures. Drug stockouts and patient complaints continued (Suarez 2010), and in 2010, America's Public Broadcast Service did a special on the shortage of HIV treatment in Mozambique (PBS Newshour 2010). Decentralization was handled poorly in Mozambique. Making the appropriate connections between what happened and other forces, possibly ones too strong for Mozambique's AIDS activists to fight, begs delving into the "theory" of decentralization promoted by authorities and experts—where it came from, what it did, and how it was made manifest in this country.

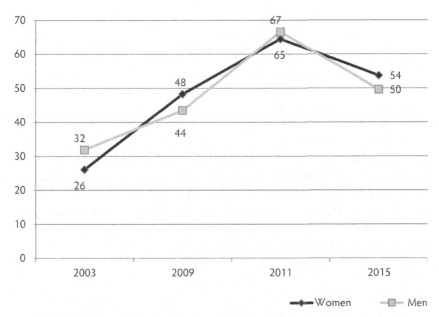

FIGURE 5.5. Percentages of women and men age fifteen to forty-nine years old who know that HIV can be transmitted from mother to child by breastfeeding and that the risk of mother-to-child transmission of HIV can be reduced by the mother taking special drugs during pregnancy, Mozambique, 2003 to 2015

HEALTH SYSTEMS FLATTENING: THE FAILED PROMISES OF DECENTRALIZATION

The day hospital closures were, in more ways than one, in total lockstep with changes occurring in other developing nations at the time. Health policy experts and scholars were actively debating the advantages and disadvantages of policies related to the administration of HIV care that emphasized the strengthening of national health systems over and above the continued implementation of piece-meal projects. Termed "health systems strengthening" (HSS), examples of folding disease-specific interventions into national health systems came primarily from the Latin American setting, where programs addressing bilharzia, maternal and child health, immunizations, vaccines, and malaria were gauged for how well their funding might better be put to use in the public domain (Rabkin and Nishtar 2011).

Given the overwhelming amount of money being spent on HIV/AIDS—which garnered about U.S.$15 billion in the first decade of the 2000s alone (El-Sadr et al. 2011)—metaphorical votes were being cast in the published literature for how well this might work in the world of HIV/AIDS. The winners of this debate emphasized the futility of short-term goals—even before all evidence in strict support of the position was available from real-world settings (Atun et al. 2010)—and insisted that funneling HIV/AIDS resources into fewer funding streams would yield better results than the continuation of fractured, small-scale efforts operating in isolation or in tandem with one other. "Horizontal" funding, with resources dedicated more to government coffers than anyplace else, was deemed more effective than "vertical" funding, or resources dedicated to smaller projects in fewer locales (Lawn et al. 2008).

Decision-makers at the WHO, the World Bank, the U.S. government, and UNAIDS decided—as we saw in the case of Mozambique—that victory in the fight against HIV lay in the hands of empowered and emboldened national health systems, not with handfuls of NGOs who bypass local structures altogether. HIV-related interventions would be unable to progress, and would ultimately be unsustainable, without addressing the systemic challenges common to the environments in which programs and health care staff found themselves. Building up the "crumbling core" of health services and facilities in developing nations, many began to argue, should be the top priority (Loewenson and McCoy 2004).

This was, in many ways, a revisit of some very old and even heated exchanges on whether it is better to fund one disease or fight them all simultaneously, whether it is best to implement "primary health care" or "selective primary health care" in postcolonial, poverty-stricken, and even war-torn states in southern Africa (Walsh and Warren 1979; Newell 1988). The difference between these strategies, when they were being considered in the late twentieth century, was their potential for different kinds of distortions. Successes associated with a rapid deployment of clinicians and staff or pouring money into quick technological fixes—such as insecticide spraying to kill mosquitoes that spread malaria—had to be weighed against the possibility that local-level processes might continue to degrade alongside them.

Yet empowering a nation could also mean lower quality or an even slower response. Governments already struggling with chronic infrastructure and logistical issues—such as being able to maintain a cold chain for vaccine storage and delivery—might only be capable of targeting basic health care issues, useful at the population level but not so much against epidemics or during spikes in the incidence of more virulent and deadly diseases. Tension around the continuing operation of Mozambican day hospitals was, subsequently, marked by very similar concerns. If we consider the facilities only as places for the distribution of pills, then of course, folding them into the main hospitals makes sense—especially from the detached perspective of planners and managers.

However, in the developed world—the United States, Europe, and other nations in the global north—there are no prohibitions against specialty clinics or programs tailored to serve vulnerable populations. These are hallmarks of administrative sophistication, not threats to the system. If the U.N., the WHO, or another managing body tried to force a highly industrialized and well-resourced

nation to "integrate" its cancer units or children's hospitals, there would be outrage. Weeding out institutes or foundations that supported them—as was happening to humanitarian NGOs throughout Mozambique—would be judged as
illogical or even illegal.

But in the majority of settings, serving or targeting a population in need is
considered a charitable mission, both to the group itself and to the rest of the
health care system. It allows providers to filter services and focus on illnesses
that cause disproportionate suffering. It decongests other facilities so that a basic
level of care can continue unhindered for everybody else and gives specialists
opportunities they otherwise wouldn't have to hone their craft. This logic, that
disease-specific clinics are appropriate and progressive, also holds true from the
perspective of patients.

Supporting persons at higher risk for being lost to the system or remaining
invisible is typically a praiseworthy pursuit, even if such efforts do separate or
wall them off from the outside world. Providing special and at-risk persons with
their own spaces is not uncommon. Leibing and Cohen (2006) note how the
culture of nursing homes, in the case of dementia sufferers, supports creative
expression and selfhood among the aging. Janovicek (2007) portrays women's
shelters as homes away from home, spots where women can recuperate and
begin to reconstruct their lives after episodes of domestic abuse. Glasser (2010),
studying soup kitchens, notes the sense of community that homeless persons
developed there, which served a greater purpose than just providing basic meals.
Clients developed resilience to personal crises through the development of
social capital and networks of support. Targeted services, clinical or otherwise,
do not have to be a burden, and dismantling them is less, rather than more, likely
to strengthen a health system.

Specialized services are typical of a well-developed health system, and there
are some very practical reasons for it. The therapeutic landscape of a clinic
serving a vulnerable population, or a specific illness, carries with it a clear
health promotion message and social functions. It can be designed to attract
them and keep them coming back (Curtis et al. 2007). The integration of peer
support—as in mental-health or drug-addiction treatment (Wilton and Deverteuil 2006)—becomes more possible. "Personhood" is better sustained as clients are more able to confront and manage issues that apply only to them and
not others (McLean 2007). Day hospitals embodied all this, and so, for many
Mozambican activists and HIV-positive patients, their "decentralization" bor-
dered on injustice. For them, this was not a sophisticated theory of third-world
health care; it was another word for "defunding."

During a visit to Pemba on September 6, 2009, just days before the protest, the president of MONASO (responsible for doling out funding to AIDS
associations) had a sit-down meeting with association members from Pemba

City and surrounding areas. Her monologue centered on the falling budget of the organization. As NGOs began to "hand over" more and more duties to the government, MONASO had become increasingly responsible for financially maintaining most of the AIDS associations. It was becoming unsustainable. She criticized AIDS associations for being artificial. "Especially these newer associations," the director explained, "they have a tendency to appear and then disappear. Their existence depends on whether or not we give them money. When we don't, they stop functioning." She complained that NGOs were shoveling their responsibilities for some AIDS associations onto MONASO and stated that the problem was "decentralization." This was the result of the *crise financeira* (financial crisis), she indicated, pointing to the global economic recession of 2008 and 2009. She then told everybody—this was the point of her visit—that MONASO would not be able to support all the associations in the way it had before.

Activists who had worked directly for MONASO would be dismissed (though there really weren't very many). MONASO would cease to print the books, brochures, and pamphlets that were previously distributed in order to educate people on HIV/AIDS prevention and relevant legislation. Instead, those groups that had computers would have to download and print them on their own. "This should give the groups more pride," she told us, "because they will be acting more independently." In addition, attendance at MONASO's annual elections would be slimmed down. Only one activist from each province would be chosen to go instead of the usual five.

This and other encounters with coordinators in charge of HIV projects and programs in the country began to convince activists that the word *decentralization* signified defunded and broken budgets. Another example involved funding for the December 1 World AIDS Day celebrations that year, in 2009. Pemba's Núcleo indicated that the budget had been cut by more than half, from U.S.$12,000 in 2008 to U.S.$4,800, also because of what they termed "decentralization." The term became synonymous with lack of funding, unemployment for activists, and diminished opportunities in the city's HIV/AIDS sector.

At the opposite extreme, the mainstream literature on HIV/AIDS uses the term decentralization very differently. Rather than being synonymous with defunding, it is often found alongside helpful sounding words like "integration," "health systems," and "strength":

> By placing emphasis on strengthening district-level health systems to provide integrated primary care, the tools [offered in this guidebook] result in improved patient referral, case management and communication between levels of the health system. Strong involvement of people living with HIV as expert patients during training and their participation in clinical teams as community health

workers supports effective chronic care. The *decentralization* of services to the community level provides services close to home, supports family-based care and empowers patient self-management. Such community-based approaches to health service delivery not only help to overcome geographical distances but also address social distances by ensuring that health services are *responsive to the needs of the community*. (WHO 2009: 119; my emphasis)

Similar excerpts are ubiquitous in official assessments of decentralization, a term that, despite its significance to HSS, has a turbulent, even scandalous, history.

As the word for a process not at all new in Africa (Muhumuza 2008), decentralization in its classical form refers to the devolution of power to lower levels of government (so addressing the needs of the community). Applied to politics, decentralization harkens to participatory democracy (Kenworthy 2014), intended to spread autonomy and accountability. Based on the principle of subsidiarity, in theory, decentralization promotes greater decision-making by deferring matters to the lowest, most competent authority. In an abstract way, this came across as a very good idea in the 1980s and '90s, as part of World Bank efforts to get African countries to take responsibility for their own development (Abrahamsen 2004; Thörn 2016).

In reality, attempts to undertake such reforms on the political spectrum manifested as structural adjustment programs, aimed toward bringing about a lean and efficient state that could promote privatization, business, and global capitalism (Ferguson 1994). While political decentralization and HSS appear on the surface to differ, they overlap in the belief that benefits flow primarily from efficiency. They also always promise these benefits in the future, conveniently ignoring misalignment between "good" theory and eventual "bad" outcomes— a consequence of decentralization that did not go unnoticed in Pemba.

From the perspective of most patients in Pemba, decentralization was a very disruptive thing. MONASO was going to stop funding their associations because of decentralization. The pharmacy, waiting area, and even lay activists who worked closely with them, were all taken away when their day hospital was closed, also because of decentralization. Many patients—as I am about to describe in the next section—stopped coming for treatment and found medication more difficult to obtain. Experts writing about decentralization and HSS do not acknowledge such issues but offer these types of conclusions instead and often without providing data:

A recent subject of debate concerns the merits of vertical (targeted) versus horizontal (general) approaches to health-care provision. Although a disease-specific, targeted approach has increased access to ART for millions of individuals worldwide, increasing emphasis is now being placed on general investment in health care systems, infrastructure, and human resources to address a broader spectrum of diseases. *Decentralization* of access to health services, with a shift towards community-based care and task-shifting away from physicians to trained nurses and lay health care workers, has also been shown to increase access to ART and improve adherence and follow-up. (Barlett and Shao 2009: 638; my emphasis)

Such statements, made prior to and during the HDD closures in Mozambique, were poor predictors of current realities. As previously noted, although the sheer number of people on ART in Mozambique is higher, retention has gotten worse, dropping from 56 to 40 percent (MISAU 2017a).

Top-down, influential institutions like UNAIDS agreed, however, that decentralization was "the key factor" in improving patient retention and various forms of adherence support—including that of support groups (2013: 21). Mozambique is singled out in such assessments, which claim that "all African countries are successfully decentralizing" their ART services (38). Voices from the field, however—like Dr. Decroo of MSF, who was present at the closure of Tete day hospital—noted that the decentralization efforts in Mozambique were hampered by a lack of infrastructure, shortages of human resources, organizational challenges, and drug shortages (Decroo et al. 2014). After decentralization in that region, patient attrition under the new system approached two times that of the old one (Decroo et al. 2009). Others with a long history of working in Mozambique—such as James Pfeiffer (2010) and his organization Health Alliance International—at first spoke out against the HDDs, portraying them as NGO creations. Later, after seeing that decentralization was carried out too quickly and the government wasn't prepared, he and his team suggested that some of the day hospitals should have remained open (Lambdin et al. 2013).

That was undoubtedly the case because relative to other health clinics in Mozambique, HDDs were veritable centers of excellence. They embodied the very same creative approaches that many proponents of decentralization now recommend enacting. These are portrayed as new ideas, distinctive, and innovative but were already happening in the HDDs at the time of their closures. Bedelu and colleagues (2007) suggested that decentralizing services enabled "task shifting," or the use of lower-level health care workers and lay "adherence counselors" to cater to higher numbers of patients in South Africa. Day hospitals already did this, however, by using health technicians to prescribe ARVs and perform assessments and activists to educate new patients and fill out forms. Bemelmans and colleagues (2010) point out that in Malawi, creating "health surveillance assistants" to work in "improved health posts" allowed HIV-positive patients to be seen separately and faster than in the main hospital. Day hospitals were already separate, faster facilities, "improved" posts for HIV care. Long and colleagues (2011) praised Johannesburg's Crosby Clinic for building a separate waiting area, consultation rooms, and pharmacy for HIV-positive patients independent of other clinic services.

Day hospitals already had each of these features. Nearly everything that expert authors identified as goals and objectives for decentralization to strive for and achieve had previously been undertaken in the HDDs as a matter of design. Yet their disappearance and devolution went unnoticed in most mainstream publications, particularly the reports of multinational institutions. Out of the forgetfulness that resulted, by now in 2017, recommendations have come full circle. A recently published analysis of ART in Mozambique calls, yet again, for using patients as adherence counselors in clinics (Auld et al. 2016)—something that was already happening in most HDDs prior to decentralization.

While it was never possible to upgrade all government clinics to the level of the HDDs, keeping some or all of them open as the government took on more responsibility would have made more logistical sense. Likely, this was less of a concern than some other factors. For instance, 2009 was an election year in Mozambique. It's possible that the government wanted to appear in charge and capable of caring for its citizens over and above the perceived incursions of international NGOs into the health sector. Closing HDDs allowed the government both to save face domestically and to cater to changing international trends. Moreover, there may have been financial inspiration for closing the HDDs.

"Performance-based financing" (PBF) is an increasingly influential trend in southern Africa (Gergen et al. 2017), one that has gained traction since the World Bank began heavily funding such schemes in 2008—the same year Mozambique started closing down HDDs. PBF involves cash payments to health centers, providers, and sometimes even patients, tying rewards to "indicators," including (for example) the number of beneficiaries served, number of staff trained, number of successful live births, or number of persons placed on ART. In this data-driven approach, facilities report their results via forms and websites, which are tabulated and monitored from afar in order to determine how well the clinic or hospital is functioning and meeting demands. Without state "ownership," clinics and patients outside governmental records are less likely to "count,"[11] diverting possible funding and credit for successful responses or interventions.

While there is no outright indication that the HDD closures were PBF inspired, scholars have noted that HSS programs and PBF schemes are comingled, especially in Africa (Paul et al. 2017; Soeters et al. 2011; Bucagu et al. 2012). They share the same "building blocks": health service delivery, health workforce, health information systems, access to essential medicines, health systems financing, and leadership and governance (Suthar et al. 2017; WHO 2010). This convergence is intentional. The six building blocks help determine the formulas that determine the checklists used to allocate conditional cash payments both to patients (who exhibit good behavior) and to workers in national health systems.

While HSS remains somewhat hazily defined, in the popular imagination, it clearly alludes to empowering the state (Mercer, Thompson, and de Araujo 2014). PBF, in comparison, is less well understood. One published overview defines PBF as a "black box" (Renmans et al. 2016), reliant on complex data systems and outside verification agents. Another study complicates PBF as in flux, seeking to design "optimal" and "interconnected" contracts among different actors within and outside of the health system (Paul and Renmans 2017).

At least two major concerns arise from the overlap between PBF and HSS. First, financial incentives are associated with higher performance, which is more easily measured in terms of quantity rather than quality. This allows donors to continue to pursue their own agendas by rewarding certain priority indicators and still excluding the state and patients as decision-makers. Second, because PBF is primarily contracts based, the perceived benefits of working through the state instead of NGOs raises the same old concerns about inefficiency and complexity but on the administrative side. Instead of the duplication of service provision, there is a duplication of resources for data monitoring and audits. Instead of health workers being drawn to higher paying employment opportunities with NGOs, incentives put in place through PBF impact wages and motivations in different but equally uncertain ways. Even as PBF converges with HSS, reliant as it is on contracts and new sorts of partners and experts, it does not resolve local problems of ineffective communication, inadequate infrastructure, or good management required to enact lasting changes in developing national health systems (Ogundeji et al. 2016).

In Mozambique, PBF is associated with a U.S.$100 million HSS project in Gaza and Nampula Provinces, under PEPFAR contractor EGPAF.[12] A PBF-related scheme is also credited with improving performance of Mozambique's Central Medical Store, responsible for managing pharmaceutical procurement in the country (Spisak et al. 2016).[13] These developments indicate that outside technical and financial assistance play no less of a role in Mozambique's health sector than before. HSS—especially in light of PBF—may not increase sovereignty and decision-making at the state level but may perpetuate preexisting or underlying power structures. Examining HSS in Mozambique requires looking beyond the narrow outputs of numbers and indicators to whose goals are being actively pursued, entirely reframing the initial debate around vertical and horizontal programs. Rather than catering to patients' needs, the continuing convergence of state and donor interests may sufficiently explain HSS. Rather than promoting robust, flexible health systems, HSS may support rudimentary, easily monitored ones instead.

Nevertheless, HSS is highly regarded as necessary and ethical. The most well-funded and influential bodies and entities—the World Bank, the WHO, UNAIDS—have thrown their full weight behind the implementation of HSS and decentralization policies. HSS has been firmly placed on the agenda of every single global health initiative operating in developing countries, including PEP-FAR, the Global Fund, the Global AIDS Vaccine Alliance, and the Gates Foundation (Hafner and Shiffman 2013). Also supporting the moniker of health systems strengthening are various peer-reviewed articles (Mussa et al. 2013), government contractors (Abt Associates Inc. 2012; FHI 360 2016), think-tank analysts, and white papers presented, for example, at World Economic Forum meetings (Sekhri 2006).

Such consensus indicates an almost total shift in global health away from humanitarian assistance toward official development aid—essentially, a new "stage" of international public health (Birn 2009). Although good effort has been made to gauge the fidelity of influential actors toward HSS and its building blocks (Storeng 2014) and to police progress and levels of commitment from large funders (Warren et al. 2013), less attention has been paid to HSS and its outcomes, like the closure of HDDs. Aligning with unilateral state interests, increasing the presence and influence of GHIs, reducing diversity in health care and options for patients, these outcomes could be construed not as empowering but as "flattening" effects. Health systems strengthening, if it doesn't strengthen, turns around upon itself to become "health systems flattening."

The concept of "flattening" describes the incorporation of marginalized societies into the process of globalization (Friedman 2005). Used optimistically, "flattening" embraces the free flow of information and a rising tide of collaboration and interconnectedness. Health systems flattening acknowledges that this process can be incomplete or unfulfilling. It refers to the grooming of health systems in developing nations to be more open to capital markets. This occurs through the culling of services provided by humanitarian NGOs, making health systems less beholden to charity and more subject to the private sector. Health systems flattening takes into account worsening or flat-lined statistics at the national level (see figures 5.2 through 5.5), calling into question the adequacy of HSS as a reorganizing principle.

Part of the "flat world" desired by global elites includes health sectors that meet minimum standards and expectations. In HSS, this is imposed through data analytics, public-private partnerships, and performance-based financing to ensure conformity. Outside of predefined targets—such as those put forth in Millennium or Sustainable Development Goals—a flattened health system has no need for specialty clinics like HDDs. Pursuing a flat world entails removing them and presenting this as a cost-effective move and moral imperative.

Because of the HDD closures, the lasting effects of decentralization and HSS hit AIDS activists particularly hard. The AIDS associations continued for a brief time afterward, but many ART patients were immediately dispossessed. What happened in Pemba, and in some other cities in Mozambique, with the closure of the day hospitals qualifies for what Dear and Wolch (1987) call a "landscape of despair." Drawing on theories of therapeutic landscapes (Bell et al. 1999) human geographers have cited other examples of what happens when high numbers of service-dependent populations are discharged from programs and facilities in the name of relocating them. Communities often ascribe more stigma to facilities that cater to high-risk groups than do the groups themselves. Burnett and Moon (1983) document this in the context of hostels for the homeless in urban America. When beneficiaries are dispersed from places they frequent and consider their own, the effect is one of instability, dismantlement, and reconfiguration. It tends to disorient people, negatively impact their identity, and cause them to feel abandoned.

Official processes like these usually rely on variables that turn out to be poor surrogates for equity and fairness—like minimizing distances between services and users or maximizing the number of recipients. If intentional, this can lead to a "planned shrinkage" (Wallace 1990), a downgrading of services as communities of patients get deconcentrated and fractured and lose their collective voice. In landscapes of despair, patients are unceremoniously "dumped" onto smaller facilities—like rural clinics in Mozambique now expected to offer ART—less capable of addressing complex issues or organizing effectively to demand resources from the state.

In the case of HIV-positive patients, and from the point of view of those threatened by activism, this was very effective because it took away political power—the "master frame" of demanding universal treatment. Consequently, it also delegitimized the HIV treatment movement in the eyes of the international community. If the goal of the state is the same as the activists, to get as many people on treatment in as many places as possible, then the state is in the right not only to shut down HDDs but also to ignore and even shut down projects and programs for activists as well. This is, in part, why complaints about day hospital closures, legitimized because of "theory" and rubber-stamped by expert consensus for widespread deployment and implementation, went unacknowledged in wider circles.

But there are also other reasons this happened. HIV treatment activism was always peripheral in Mozambique and, at least in Pemba, a good example of the few exercising power over the many. It was inorganic, a garden that was not well tended. HIV treatment activism there was just one of many other industries, a job opportunity and way to get employed. The role of advocate was easily exploited, even if it arose in legitimate contexts. This meant that when the time came to call upon "activists," they were few and far between. They had to be manipulated, or organized, to stand up and represent what were supposedly the universal values of treatment activism as a social movement.

In this next section, I will describe how this was done in Pemba, unfortunately mostly through Luisa, Caridade's vice-president. Going back in time, to just before the Pemba protests happened, we see her primary role as community organizer but also main beneficiary of resources and prestige. AIDS associations hadn't completely disappeared but began to sense this would happen. The next section reveals the importance of the protests but also the frailty of the activist community in Mozambique. To understand what was changing in the health system, ART patients needed help from activists but well before it was first received. AIDS activists needed the support of more patients but hadn't properly included them in their circles. Scrambling to stay relevant after the HDD closures, association leaders like Luisa capitalized on this lack of clarity, emphasizing poor communication and patient dissatisfaction. This anxious and rebellious energy, while clearly available, wasn't well harnessed. Activists would have done better to consider smarter options for moving forward than simply protests, which turned out to be a misplaced form of resistance that was neither substantial nor effective.

As scholars of social movements have noted (Ancelovici 2015), the study of protests alone can yield substandard conclusions. The HDD protests did not signify solidarity so much as desperation but without the right ethnographic data or legwork, analysts could easily miss this point. In this next section, I will explain how Luisa positioned herself for success regardless of other outcomes, undermining the very same protests that she led and organized. My conclusions are situated along the lines of earlier assessments. Activism—like any other resource in Mozambique—is usable, expendable, potentially controversial, and subject to exploitation. Making sure it remains available and accessible to all who need it is a task or chore that deserves greater attention in the future. Meaningful activism is a precious commodity, which may need special protection to be guarded from such exploitation.

"SLACKTIVISM" AND RABBLE-ROUSING IN NORTHERN MOZAMBIQUE

"It is already done," said Dr. Saúde. "The integration has happened. There is no way to change it, and what can we do now? The government é nosso pai [is our father], and we must respect our father." Addressing the association called Esperanca da Vida at their usual meeting place on the wooden benches behind Pemba's former day hospital, Dr. Saúde, the health technician, was referring to the recent closure of the facility. "Integration" was the nicest way of putting it; a total mess was closer to the truth. I hadn't been to the HDD in a while. It was never really a calm place, but it was relatively private, protected by a high wall shielding it from view of the street. One could usually at least find a seat. Now it was overflowing with people, and it was loud. I had to force my way through the queue formed at the narrow entrance and beg pardon for disturbing people to get into the compound. I could see why ART patients were complaining; it appeared as if their hospital had been taken over by outsiders. I sat down next to the doctor.

"We have to make our own solutions," Dr. Saúde continued, "because this is a problem that needs to be confronted and dealt with." He turned toward me. "Cristiano, what do you think?" he asked. I explained what I had heard about this in other cities in Mozambique—Tete and Chimoio for example—that the changes were implemented quickly and that both staff and patients were caught off guard. I read online that patients had been complaining about having to wait in the same areas of the hospital with other patients because their health cards were green and not blue. When they presented themselves in a queue or to the staff, others noticed this and it caused anxiety and fear. "Change the color of the cards, OK," said Dr. Saúde, writing something on paper. "What else?" he looked around at the group. Somebody suggested that we needed to educate people on the virus—the default response to such inquiries. Another member said that everyone should be in the same queue and that it is perfectly normal for patients to be seen by the same doctors. "No," one woman disagreed, "a nurse who doesn't know about HIV could say it is the same thing as malaria! That it is *igual* [equal]!"

At this, everyone in the group burst out laughing, Dr. Saúde included. "She said it is *igual*!" he said, catching everybody's eye and inciting an additional round of laughter. "Look, the problem is," he continued, "that already people have stopped coming. Normally we have fifty patients per day in the day hospital. Yesterday there were three, the day before that there were only two. My bosses want to know what is happening, and they want a report. What can I tell them?"

An association member, a middle-aged man, said that "the ones who are scared are not us, but those outside of the association. They fear being discriminated against when they are in the same room with nonpositives."

Dr. Saúde turned to me and said, "What's going to happen in this country is, we are going to reach a phase where nobody gets a test, there will be no CD4 counts, we will just write a prescription for triomune and hand it to the patient and say 'here it is, go and get it.'"

Esperanca da Vida was an association composed of all ART patients, about twenty-five people. Many had been to Maputo and "trained" to carry out home-based care, but nobody did. There were no salaries and no spaces for them in formal projects. All they had was a charcoal-making business and a chicken coup. The group said it was waiting for the DREAM program—the Maputo-based NGO initiative that funded their training—to build them a nutrition center in Pemba so they could get free food. Some of the group's members joined Esperanca da Vida because they didn't like the way Caridade was being managed. They were particularly critical of Luisa, Caridade's vice-president, for not sharing information with them and for kicking some of them out of their paid positions as workers for UNICEF, Action Aid, or other NGOs.

Knowing this about the group, I was surprised to see Luisa herself turn the corner of the building and comfortably sit down next to Dr. Saúde. He was expecting her, and after greeting everybody, she launched into what was apparently her assigned lecture topic—*associativismo* and leadership—even more important now that AIDS associations were losing their HDDs. Luisa began by explaining that the group needed to have an organogram and that only the president and the vice-president can sign checks or authorize a dispersal of money. She went on to explain that Caridade had been so successful that HIV patients in Cabo Delgado were not as behind the times as they used to be, that they were more organized, and cited Caridade's activities in other towns and districts as evidence of the association's success. "We are known at the national level," she bragged, and offered Esperanca da Vida membership in RENSIDA, Mozambique's national people with AIDS umbrella association.

I was surprised to hear this suggestion. Just a few days before, having beers with Luisa in the front yard of her house, she told me that she had RENSIDA *nas palma das mãos* (in the palm of her hands). She didn't seem keen on sharing her privileges with others. Her frequent trips to Maputo for trainings and her position as coordinator of a UNICEF program were extremely lucrative for her. She rarely showed up at Caridade's office but was still somehow the first point of contact whenever someone important arrived in Pemba and wanted to discuss the human rights of HIV-positive patients in the city. The latest example of this involved a researcher from the U.N. who we heard wanted to interview Caridade members about gender equality. We waited around the office all day only to find out she never left Luisa's house and departed from the Pemba airport after talking to her but not to anyone else in the group.

Plenty of Caridade members were upset with Luisa—they considered her lazy and a thief—but there was little they could do about it. Her phone number topped the list in Maputo of people to call in Pemba, and most of the group's reports passed through her hands before going on to RENSIDA. With President Antonio spending most of his days drunk, Luisa had commandeered power over Caridade, the association with the longest history of partnerships and coalition-building in the province. Luisa, after encouraging the members of Esperanca da Vida to open a group bank account, invited them to a meeting that was about to happen to plan the protest against day hospital closures in Pemba, to take place a few weeks later.

Through her Maputo contacts, Luisa became de facto leader over the Pemba protest as well. Far away from Maputo, activists in Pemba and Cabo Delgado Province had infrequent contact with others throughout the country. The organizers of the protest, the *Liga Contra Discriminação*, had been relying on her organizational abilities to ensure the widespread involvement of as many AIDS associations and patients as possible. Over the course of planning the protest, when the Maputo-based activists flew in to Pemba for meetings, Luisa was the locally appointed representative and did the most talking. In closed-door meetings with members of the *Liga*, Luisa managed to gain access over the protest's resources—boxes of "HIV Positive" T-shirts, crates of bottled water, bags of snacks, such as potato chips and cookies.

Later, we found she had sold some of these items in the markets—including the T-shirts—and there was not enough for the protesters during the march. She appointed members of her own family and friends as liaisons and persons responsible for various jobs before the protest. Her brother was to contact the police and the city council. Her mother would inform the radio station and NGOs in town. There were per diems, small amounts of money, available for these jobs. Her father would facilitate the purchase of gasoline for the motorcycles, including his own. She also decided who would carry the banners and the money spent on the materials needed to construct them. It was also decided—between Luisa and the group of activists from Maputo—that she would be the one to hand over the letter to the provincial health director on the day of the protest. Luisa had succeeded in dominating the entire process of planning for the September 11, Pemba-based march. She had become the "African big man" (Cabassi and Wilson 2005), capable of circumventing AIDS civil society in Pemba. Her reliance on her friends and family is typical of the clientelistic relationships based in the "primordial public" that Ekeh (1975) discusses in his seminal work on this topic.

Regardless, Luisa and the *Liga* tapped into some very real concerns that patients had over the loss of their day hospitals. Luisa did a fine job of identifying speakers for the larger meetings who could rile up the crowd and elicit the kind of reaction appropriate for a political protest against perceived governmental injustice. At the Red Cross building in Pemba, several activists, including Luisa, gave their testimonies in preparation for the final day. After viewing a video of the August protests, of patients marching in the streets with their T-shirts and signs through closed-off city streets, and of the clip when César of MATRAM read the grievance letter to Ivo Garrido on the steps of the Ministry of Health, Luisa stood in front of the group of about two hundred HIV-positive patients and said, "The bosses are abusing us, and it is the personal problem of Ivo Garrido. Many people already arrive late for treatment, and many think that treatment doesn't exist. This disease can't be treated like all of the others, it requires treatment for life. The patient has a right to the information they need for taking ARVs properly. And why does South Africa have special treatment centers for patients but here in Mozambique we must close them?"

Another activist (Saimon, a policeman), and one of the founding members of Caridade, followed, telling the crowd, "I was the first person on treatment in Pemba City. In the old days, we could come only one day of the week to get ARVs, but the old nurses were good. We are going back to how it was before, with limited services, only now the nurses treat us badly. There are other people who haven't been back to the hospital since this happened. If we lost people before, we're losing even more now." Cristova, another ART patient, focused on a common complaint among ART patients, the rumor that rich people did not have to wait in line at the hospital and that they had their own "night hospitals" where they could receive their treatment in secret. He said, "The problem here is discrimination, discrimination against poor people! Where are the ministers of parliament getting their treatment? Why do I never see the bosses in line at the hospital? The night hospitals are still open. We are all HIV positive but in different economic classes. We must march and show our force like patients did in Maputo."

As the meeting drew to a close, three more people took a stand, pledging their commitment to the cause of protest. These Pemba residents and ART patients were normally cut off from mainstream AIDS activism in Mozambique, but the level of their passion was tangible. Without the Liga's influence, they would have remained in the dark about why the HDD had shut down and with no direction about how to address it. Such an occurrence like this gathering was new but indicated the possible depth of civil society. Unfortunately, the Liga, an outside organization, had to facilitate it, and a cause or a threat—the loss of day hospitals—was necessary for unity.

After the meeting was over, other patients approached me with additional statements. One unnamed man, who I'd never met before, told me:

I travel here from Mieze [about twenty kilometers away]. It costs forty meticais [U.S.$1.50]. Before, I could come in the morning and get my medications quickly, even do lab tests. Now I have to wait four hours before I can go back into the hospital for the results. These medications [he shows me his prescription for an antibiotic, B vitamins, and acetaminophen] will cost me 300 meticais [about U.S.$13] in Farmácia Nova [a private pharmacy in Pemba]. I have severe headaches all day for the past week and a terrible stomachache. If I can't get my analysis today, I have to pay again to come back tomorrow. Before, things were good, why is the government doing this to us now?

Another man, a well-dressed professor who lived and worked at the teacher's training college but hid his status from his coworkers, told me, "I was always able to get my pills at the day hospital, for years, and nobody ever knew that I went there. Two days ago, I was seen in the hospital, and now I am writing letters to my boss to explain why I should be able to continue teaching even with this condition. I didn't expect this, and I may have to get a lawyer. If I get fired, I am thinking of writing my story to put in the newspaper, but I do not know where I am going to live if that happens."

I was surprised to discover some people believed that Pemba's day hospital shut down because of construction that was going on there. They had no idea it was a nationwide, government change until they attended the meeting. One man, an ART patient, said to me, "I thought that if there was more space [on the hospital's grounds], we could have continued with the separation. I had no idea any of this was happening, talking about policies and rights! All I knew was that the doctors and nurses were gone. Now, hearing about this discrimination against us, I don't know why it has been kept secret and nobody from the government told us about this." Clearly, things had gone wrong in the decentralization process. Some people weren't getting the proper medications or lab tests. Others had their positive status disclosed inadvertently. Others were entirely unaware the changes were planned at the national level. Slightly better planning could have prevented these mishaps and confusion.

The *Liga's* intent was to influence patients to march, correct misinformation, and create a united front. Yet I've already described the disappointment and what happened during the protest and afterward. Nothing changed for these ART patients. By most accounts, treatment access got even worse than it was before. The political "action" taken on the part of the *Liga* in Pemba—the protest against the day hospital closure—was fruitless for most of the province's patients. It was, however, profitable for Luisa and a few others. I will comment more on this soon. For now, let's conceive of the day hospital protests not as earth-shattering events but as minor acts of support for the cause of treatment activism.

Analyzing the concept of "slacktivism," Kristofferson, White, and Peloza (2014) note how "token acts of support" of a socially observable nature moderate later involvement in a cause. In this study, individuals who engaged in *public* support for a particular cause were less likely to meaningfully respond to follow-up requests, as compared with those who engaged in *private* support for the same exact cause. The reason had to do with self-consistency and the alignment of values. In publicly observable settings, motivations were more likely to be inspired by impression-management concerns. For individuals interested in being viewed by others, public support for a cause satisfied the criteria for their involvement. They were no more likely to support the cause in the future than those who did not initially support it at all.

Conversely, for those whose involvement with a cause was done in private, values were more likely to be derived from individual attitudes and reasoning and less prone to social influence. In these cases, subsequent involvement with a cause was more likely to remain consistent, the distance between the self and the cause was diminished, and misalignment between belief and action became aversive. In other words, reliable and persistent activism depended on personal commitment, not obvious, outward behaviors. Combating "slacktivism"—an eventual decline in support for a cause, even after high initial interest—means that values displayed to the world must first be instilled in private. For HIV patients, where both forums are essential for the cause as a whole, this suggests the need not for more protests or public displays of demands and grievances but for strong, locally situated support groups capable of voicing and consolidating their views among one another prior to airing them on the street or in the media.

While initial views on "slacktivism" stem from the online world—of consumers "clicking" the "like" buttons on Facebook pages or retweeting within the hashtags of activist Twitter accounts—in the "offline" world of Mozambique, the Liga's sudden appearance in Pemba as organizers of dissent is metaphorically similar. The need for Maputo-based activists to come to the area and fill a gap in knowledge, about the policies of the government and the rights of HIV-positive people, indicates an arbitrary relationship between the signifier and the signified, between politically savvy AIDS activists from the capital city and those who are less aware, comparatively lost on the nation's northern shore and of limited interest to central government. For them, marching in a protest is clicking on the "like" button—a token act of support not likely to develop much further due to foundational lack of initial involvement. Commercializing a protest, the "social marketing" of activism and human rights, is likely unsustainable and unlikely to lead to subsequent meaningful action, especially if not enough attention was paid to the groundwork for such action previously and in private.

Unity and social solidarity, therefore, remain elusive, made up, in need of a crafted defense. For the Maputo protests to be reproduced and restaged in other parts of the country is also to treat ART patients not primarily as brothers and sisters for a cause but as consumers of a model or brand that needed distribution and publicity. Even though it hooked in to organic complaints, the public platform of rabble-rousing was unavailable in the ordinary medium of Mozambican activism without encouragement from idealists and gatekeepers. When the activists of Esperanca da Vida were asking along with Dr. Saúde, "What do we do now that the integration has occurred?" the answer came from Luisa and other quasi-elites with, perhaps, different or additional motives and intentions. The theme of the protests—down with stigma and discrimination—was, in the end, much too generalized to lend to any particular province, city, or group of patients. It may also have obfuscated other, more practical, locally defined terms of negotiation and retaliation, such as the need for lawyers, local AIDS centers, or private pharmacy stipends for ART patients.

What else might have occurred without this imposition of the national over the local, of the transnational over the domestic, and of the chanting and marching AIDS activist over the problem-solving capacity of particular support groups we will now never know. If any fruit grew from the protest in Pemba, Luisa consumed most of it. This situation suggests that activists who seek public recognition may engage in multiple, even contradictory roles—that of challenging neoliberal economic injustices and policies and also that of obtaining prestige promotions.

Soon after the Pemba protest, Luisa created a new AIDS association, with herself as the president. She called it *Si Peke Yangu* (I Am Not Alone) and told me that it was for women only. She invited me over for a meeting one day, which took place at her home in *Bairro Natite*. When I arrived, the women were eating chicken and drinking sodas—in Pemba, this is a special treat. Dressed in matching *capulanas*, they were practicing songs and dances for the upcoming World AIDS Day celebration on December 1. I was asked to take some pictures of them on my camera and record a video of the group on my phone. As I did, I noticed that I knew some of the women—they were Luisa's neighbors, and others were friends of hers, likely not HIV-positive. Later, I found out that the group had gotten funding from MONASO—for meals during meetings, for the *capulana* material, and even for a computer that Luisa kept in her home to write grants and reports. The pictures and video were sent to Maputo as part of a project application for a local women's HIV support group, which up until then had not existed in Pemba.

Other AIDS associations had been trying for years to get this kind of attention from MONASO. Luisa's outspokenness, her willingness to be seen and heard and talk about her illness in public, was a qualification with disproportionate benefits. At the World AIDS Day festivities, her new group sang a song for the governor, his wife, and a minister of parliament that went like this: "We are *Si Peke Yangu*, and our history is a long one." The association at that time was less than two months old.

In 2011, Luisa was hired as a project manager by RENSIDA, and left Pemba to go and work in Maputo. She continued to remain vice-president of Caridade and president of Si Peke Yangu during her absence. Her time in Maputo was short, however. She was found embezzling project funds and using RENSIDA money to support her own lifestyle in the capital. To this day, Luisa remains integral to the functioning of Caridade, but the association has slimmed down considerably. Its members now only include those who get paid for carrying out project work in Pemba's bairros. Other AIDS associations in Pemba have ceased functioning—Esperanca da Vida, Nashukuru, Ajuda à Próxima—no longer meet together or carry out project work in their villages. Bem Vindo, the home-based care group that had received EGPAF and PEPFAR funding from 2009 to 2014, continued to operate, and most of its members were not even HIV positive.

Certain other "activists" in Pemba still get visits from important people in Maputo. Recently, I came across a photo of Luisa on a social media website with the director of a major U.S. donor. The caption indicated that he was being briefed on the human rights situation of HIV-positive people in Cabo Delgado Province. Luisa's identity as an AIDS activist continues to profit her enormously. As the name *Si Peke Yangu* suggests, she is probably not alone; there may be many activists whose public and private presentations of themselves conflict and threaten to undermine or cheapen solidarity at the local level. Outsiders and visitors must work with wider bases of activists to offset this bias and to ensure that equal opportunity is given to those who may be rendered hidden or voiceless by a few strong and dominating personalities within specific activist cultures.

THE KNIFE IN A GUNFIGHT: HIV TREATMENT ACTIVISM AFTER HEALTH SYSTEMS STRENGTHENING

What the closing of day hospitals in Mozambique suggests is that if AIDS activism is unable to evolve—to move beyond a focus on treatment—it can, will, or may already have become irrelevant in places like Pemba. Since its inception, popular understandings of AIDS activism have centered on its capacity for performance, for theater, for pinpointing, targeting, and engaging in smear campaigns against a perceived enemy of one kind or another. This is less useful than we are often led to believe. Studying ACT UP, in the early days of American AIDS activism, Gamson (1989) draws attention to how the group's actions sometimes got noticed but at other times were completely ignored. South Africa's TAC gained immense publicity with its street theater and legal actions against the government (Nattrass 2007).

Today, however, the group finds itself amid paralyzing budget cuts, abandonment by many of its previous donors, and dropping down the political agenda in South Africa and internationally (Nicolson 2014). The question worth asking is whether or not this model—with its anger and its semimilitant approach to organizing patient demands under the auspices of political resistance—is really all that representative or transferable. Perhaps it is itself the outlier and the anomaly when compared with other, less commonly studied examples of unity and solidarity. Post health systems strengthening, treatment activism in developing nations is more impotent than ever before. It is obsolete, no longer pivotal, and a relic—the knife in a gunfight, an almost useless weapon against untouchable multinational policies promising to strengthen health systems. Moreover, the patient voice is now less, rather than more, valuable. What emerged in Mozambique is the idea that HIV patients, supposedly, are now no different than anyone else attempting to navigate the health system.[14] Ironically, the "decentralization" of day hospitals—properly executed—fits perfectly into the "master frame" of fairness and equity that was always at the center of the AIDS activist agenda.[15]

Scholars of social movements interested in "framing processes" and "collective action frames," like poor treatment access, note that they are not merely carriers of ideas or naturally occurring meanings that unexpectedly grow out of events, arrangements, or ideologies. They are, instead, relied upon by "movement actors" and viewed by them as "signifying agents" (Benford and Snow 2000: 613). From this perspective, AIDS activists, like members of any other social movement, actively engage in the production of meaning—in its generation, diffusion, and functionality and the way in which it operates among other members and within the movement itself. There is intention here. Goals and objectives are set and pursued. There is, therefore, also responsibility and culpability. The actions, claims, and demands of AIDS activists in the past were, in essence, tantamount to preauthorization for this international trend toward strengthening health systems in developing nations.

Even though consent was not explicitly obtained from every ART patient in Pemba for the closure of their day hospital, those at the highest levels of governance were operating on an implicit assumption—and ultimately, it was a good one—that any complaints about "decentralization" would fall upon deaf and unsympathetic ears. The world was now convinced that HIV-positive patients are equal, despite evidence to the contrary that they are not—due to persistent stigma and threats to routine access to health care. AIDS activism, tied so intimately to notions of injustice as it relates primarily to the availability of medications, was relatively unequipped to refocus or to shift its master frame appropriately, away from a historical standard and toward other types of "therapy"—the virtue of the day hospital as, for example, a drop-in center or social club. It was unable to attack the "openness" of health systems strengthening, its inclusivity, its appeal to a revised vision of diversity, not of HIV exceptionalism, but the human rights of everyone else—the rest of the nation's populace—in their stead.

There are a number of other ways—perhaps more effective than protests—that patients and activists could have approached the package of events described in this chapter. They could have demanded an end to all perceived "foreign" incursions into Mozambique—of PEPFAR, UNAIDS, and the WHO, in the name of "fairness" or even sovereignty. Complaints could have been made against the practices of certain community-based organizations and freshly minted contractors carrying out HIV programs in the country—the ones that the government privileged in instituting health systems strengthening. State acquiescence to donor demands and declines in HIV funding might have been laid bare. The double standard applied in this process could have been better explored, asking questions about why the government was able to retain its National AIDS Council, AIDS-specific task forces, and bureaucratic funding for targeted HIV/AIDS programs even as patient clinics and facilities were forced to shut down. Demands could have been made to incorporate funding for support groups into the framework of health systems strengthening in Mozambique, to make AIDS associations an integral part of the health system. Activists might also have critiqued the attack on small projects, in solidarity with international medical NGOs like MSF or Medicos del Mundo that also felt unduly targeted by sweeping national reforms and state demands for them to change focus.

But AIDS activism, largely writ, is unable to incorporate most of the items on this list. They are too context-specific. Limited to an obstinate form of activist orthodoxy, the only types of considerations able to make the short list—the gold standard used to unite the broadest possible base of people to its cause—concern biomedicine and the state alone. The draw toward a fight and toward war is not a feather in the cap of AIDS activism, it is a bane to its existence, a proclivity that frequently oversteps its bounds by preventing other types of dialogue.

A good deal of reshaping, remolding, reconfiguration, and even exclusionary thought is necessary to point to "valid" forms of AIDS activism and what it portends as its collective identity. The assumption—embraced and developed by political process theory and those who search for the achievement of short-term goals—is that social movements must shape public policy and state action to qualify as a force for social change. Consequently, political process theorists, in parallel with popular media, television, newspapers, and journalists, engage in a sensationalization of activism that positions the state as more powerful than it truly is—as target, audience, and arbiter of social movement demands. But the real bias, the flaw in cultural theory, is most blatant and emerges in case study selection, in the kinds of movements examined and the activities observed and explained. A protesting group alone is not good enough data. Treating it as such permits rather than inhibits "slacktivism," promoting those who seek social recognition over those who do not, threatening the long-term stability of the movement itself.

The Mozambican protests against day hospital closures did not signify the breaking open of long bottled-up tensions on the part of activists. As a political opportunity, it was short lived, a half-opened window. The protests were rushed and inorganic, exposing the unevenness of shared understandings among patients there. The protests were not liberating but constraining and confirmation of the end of an era—one where states, donors, and others invested in global health had slightly more respect for AIDS activists, their demands, and the ideas they brought to the bargaining table.

6 · BIOSOCIAL GOVERNMENTALITY

What is activism? The answer, often, is that it involves resistance and is political and empowering. Yet even as affronts against human rights inspire people to collective action, the unity that results can be fragile, and its lasting effects questionable. *Landscapes of Activism* highlights Caridade, an HIV support group that went through all the right steps to help people take control and then all the wrong steps for them to lose it. Stories like this are not commonly told in the activist world, though they are likely quite common.

Regarding an affliction or threat, *in*quisitiveness about what to do gives way to solidarity, which leads to an accumulation of hope and a feeling that the group can affect significant change. Eventually, *ac*quisitiveness, self-promotion, competition, and even aggression gain access, the consequences of which are polluting, and result in decline. Activism, or activist-ness, is not safe and secure underneath a "sacred canopy" (Berger 1990). The activist "universe"—even in the rather small corner occupied by HIV and AIDS—is made up of multiple "sets" of realities. Though the accounts of HIV patient groups differ slightly, the prevailing gist is very clear—without becoming political, they have no chance. Through the lens of Caridade, however, it's easy to see that the highest reality is not always a political one.

Outcomes of recent events spell out this surprising conclusion. Political patienthood had generally assumed the progress of a healthy activism. In the first decade of the 2000s, all signs pointed to the victory of AIDS activists—squarely arriving on the agendas of U.N. organizations, watching the fall of HIV/AIDS denialism, and seeing rebounding lifespans. Some activists might have been correct to conclude that their work was successful. Yet since then, the parameters have changed. HIV became a concern for corporations, contractors, governments, and a market industry either truly invested or masking itself behind a façade of goodwill. The watchword now is treatment, and we live under this regime. Rising numbers of infected persons and persistent problems in retaining patients in treatment programs counter the optimistic narratives of health systems strengthening and limitless biomedical intervention. Some provinces and age groups in Mozambique are now more susceptible to HIV, though the targets of focused prevention campaigns should have been realized long ago. Calls for the restoration of community priorities and of a thriving, independent civil society are now barely heard among technocratic shouts for more facilities, more experts, and wider drug distribution.

What was necessary before, or alongside all this, was rebuilding societies still in disarray from high mortality, recovering the basic requirements of a healthy citizenship, flourishing domestic lives, dignifying jobs, sound education, a deep reservoir of social support, and a broad awareness of multiple health threats. Compared with these struggles, gaining access to treatment was easy and just an initial step. Under different circumstances, it might even have happened anyway, as a basic side effect of progressing science or more substantial and enduring social solidarity. In the case of AIDS activism, as it has most distinctly been promoted and practiced, what appears to be missing is the importance of group cohesion, relationality and encounter, the consolation derived from these combinations, and the satisfaction of successfully meeting life's challenges together. In terms of theories used to grasp them, these ideas were much better encompassed in biosociality than in biological citizenship—but the latter was somehow privileged and got the most attention.

Biosociality, as first conceived by Paul Rabinow (1996), very much addressed relatedness, mutual interactions, and feelings of belonging in addition to any paths toward treatment that might emerge therein. It was intended to open up, rather than close off, the potential social interactions between humans and rare or incurable disease. Making his predictions about future biosocial "groups," Rabinow states, "These groups will have medical specialists, laboratories, narratives, traditions and a heavy panoply of pastoral keepers to help them experience, share, intervene in and 'understand' their fate" (1996: 186). For Rabinow, biosociality was a consequence of modernity and a potential catalyst for fundamental social change. The "group," however, was not just a vehicle for obtaining treatment. It was a thriving point of contact that bridged the lay-expert knowledge divide and served as a deposit for tradition, a place for sharing, and for life (or fate) to "happen."

Biological citizenship, on the other hand, with its focus on state governance and special interests, very much emphasized the rights of the group and the importance of applying pressure. While Rose and Novas (2005) spoke in general terms about a variety of health activisms to explore biological citizenship, the prism of HIV/AIDS best exemplified the shockwaves produced when one group of people (the privileged "West") had access to testing and treatment facilities, while a majority of others did not. Because collective mobilization hinged, to some degree, on raising awareness and pooling together sufferers from around the globe, the promotion of activism for purposes of agitation came to be understood as a much greater responsibility than having pleasant and productive small group meetings. This, perhaps, is how biological citizenship had a homogenizing effect on biosociality, at least in the case of HIV/AIDS—by implying activists should be more outspoken and demanding. With HIV treatment now widely available and outspokenness unnecessary to obtain it, the distortions of this trend are more evident. So too, is the notion that if biological citizenship meant staging protests and generally being disruptive, not all activists agreed with such tactics in the first place.

Many in Mozambique, for example, stood in direct tension with the idea of airing their behavior, HIV-positive status, or concerns in public. Lucinda, a nurse who once worked for RENSIDA, Mozambique's national AIDS association, expressed horror at the ideas generated by a visiting activist from the United States: "She came to my office [in Maputo] to offer us money and suggested that we fight with our government. 'Make some [picket] signs,' she told us, 'and march through the streets of the city.' She suggested that we complain about the way we were being treated. I told her that if we did that our organization would not last long. This is Mozambique, not America! I said to her that here, in Mozambique, we work *with* our government not *against* it. We don't insult others who we know will help us."

Lucinda nearly refused to grant me an interview because she'd had a bad experience with another researcher, a college student from Europe who worked with AIDS associations through a local NGO. Lucinda told me:

> When she was here, she visited with a lot of AIDS associations. She said that she wanted to ask questions, but what she really wanted was to teach them something. She spent a lot of time talking to them about what is activism. Some of the presidents from the provinces she visited complained to me, said they were embarrassed by her. "We don't want this lady telling us how to do our job," that is what they told me. She told them that good activists talk to others about their illness, that they don't hide or speak quietly, and aren't ashamed. She insulted me too, told me I was too embarrassed to share my disease status with others. I told her, "Miss, what you are going to report in your country is not going to help us."

What Lucinda's statements suggest is that "activism" is a social construct and heavily culturally influenced. Calling attention to the perhaps unconscious encroachment of Western values upon Mozambican ones exposes a dichotomy that may help contextualize the preference for a global model—one that proliferates in cosmopolitan or urban areas—over local, small-scale, culturally recognizable forms of minimizing the impact of HIV in less obvious or noteworthy ways.

As a result, many of us who write about AIDS activists have fallen into a trap, one that presumes biosociality should lead to biological citizenship and that the highest purpose of HIV patient groups is to have their demands met by outside benefactors, states, or others with more power. It is certainly the case that pharmaceuticals are a resource that most patients cannot manufacture or secure on their own, but there is more to biosociality than that captured through a focus on treatment alone. The emphasis mostly on politics, and the rather dominant version of activism that has been cast as the desirable norm, leaves much about "the group" undisclosed and undescribed.

The most prominent thesis—that progress for people with HIV depends on involvement with politics—I believe is harmful, and here, I will claim an opposite thesis. In the posttreatment era, what HIV patient groups need most is to be divorced from politics in order to remain less affected. Ideally, to be effective, the support group would be above the fray, less subject to interruptions to its development by any other actor or party, answerable to no other for its activities. It would be oriented more toward personal recovery and preventing disease relapse, toward an improvement in quality of life rather than competing for funding or working on projects promoted by NGOs.

Biosociality—a shared social consciousness or identity, with its potential to bind persons together in solidarity and combat against a threat or enemy—is relevant in its potential to create dialogue and facilitate communication. But we must be aware of how noticeable this is, especially on the part of those in power. Biosociality—describing it, documenting it, labeling it—makes people with HIV more visible. It also makes them more governable, into better identifiable targets, more directly subject to the confines of what Foucault (and many others) calls "governmentality."

My work here is preceded by many colleagues invested in the topic of HIV support groups. Like me, Ippolytos Kalofonos (2008) and Kenly Fenio (2009) entered into the field evaluating the integrity of Mozambican AIDS associations. Some of us were seeking evidence that civil society was part of the solution to the AIDS crisis. The environment at the time led to high expectations. The prevailing theory concerning AIDS activism was that suffering, caused by a lack of treatment, stimulates demand and wakes from dormancy politically active creatures that are capable, via solidarity and persistent political resistance, of obtaining what they rightly deserve from corrupt, greedy, immoral states and companies that would otherwise prefer to see them die or simply don't care. All of us, of course, problematized this algorithm. Essentially, like many theoretical constructs, it was porous and not a very good one.

Still, the fissures and cracks inherent in this myth tend to be only tangentially addressed in dissertations and full-length books in ways that short, high-impact articles overlook and do not make clear (Robins 2006; Nguyen 2007; compare with later books, Robins 2010; Nguyen 2010). The valorization of heroics, the depiction of iconic patients or groups as representative of others, as readily generalizable stand-ins and examples of best practices, cast a wide shadow over the realistic situations of the majority of patient groups in sub-Saharan Africa. The HIV support group was in very few cases an appropriate site for cultivating broader social revolution. Portraying it that way was dangerous for the groups and drowned out competing events and understandings of activists, their roles, challenges, and accomplishments.

At the root of this algorithm and presumption—that biosociality leads to biological citizenship—was the overwhelming flood of literature available about South Africa's Treatment Action Campaign; it was tempting to compare it with other groups in other places. Likely, the overemphasis on TAC had just as much to do with South Africa's middle-income status as it did with TAC's apparent successes. The nation's accessibility to researchers, widespread use of the English language, the availability of respected universities, and the primacy of business markets there are rarely factored into what was depicted as a continent-wide, even global, independent, and grassroots fight for civil and human rights. Since South Africa is also known as the protest capital of the world (Brown 2015), it's no wonder TAC grabbed so much attention, exceeding standards by fitting that mold.

However, despite some very real organizational challenges and performance issues (Marcis 2012), TAC was often portrayed as powerful, a force to be reckoned with, a model to emulate, a solid victory over racism, classism, and apartheid—a monolith: "TAC employs the political lexicon of the struggle . . . TAC events commonly start with the right-fisted salute and the cry of 'Amandla!' [power]" (Grebe 2011: 852). TAC scholars tended to conjure such images to paint the situation as a worker's fight against capitalism and medical inequality. This was partly true but uniquely South African at many junctures. TAC's supposed success impacted groups like Caridade in Mozambique in ways that were not entirely constructive. HIV patient groups that do not live up to similar expectations were more easily dismissed as ineffective and lower down on an imaginary ladder of progress than the politically successful TAC.

Scholars tended to rank African HIV patient groups according to how similar they were to TAC. Kalofonos (2008: 216) noted that "the tactics of TAC emerged out of the apartheid struggle. . . . There has never been a comparable large-scale, sustained grassroots political movement in Mozambique . . . The practices and tactics of Mozambican associations emerge out of evangelical church practices and rather than agitating for political change, these groups are more likely to seek accommodation within the status quo, and are more oriented toward daily survival." This was undoubtedly true and stems from excellent research. Still, it pointed to a bias for political upheaval, for challenges and disruptions, options that may never have been appropriate in Mozambique.

Fenio (2011: 718–722; my emphasis), a political scientist, argues that "Mozambican associations are *still* fearful of speaking out against the government . . . South Africans are most free in their ability to critique government and vocalize opposition." I emphasize the word *still* in this last quote as an indication that Mozambican patient groups are expected to do better not in terms of managing their own groups but in beginning to act more like South Africa's TAC—to not just be biosocial but become biological citizens. Ida Susser's dichotomy between "adaptive" and "transformative" activists was very similar. Patients who made and sold products for tourists on the streets of Durban were given less space in her ethnography than patients who spoke openly about their illness and attempted to recruit others into their group (Susser 2009). This selection bias was evident in much writing about AIDS activists. There was an expectation that patients conforming to a political mind, a political subjectivity, were more valuable, better off, with apparently higher potential than others.

Again from South Africa, "experiences of illness, treatment, and participation in TAC and MSF can produce radical transformations in subjectivity and identity that go well beyond conventional liberal democratic conceptions of 'rights' and 'citizenship' . . . TAC and MSF activists argue that they are not only interested in medical treatment but also concerned with creating 'empowered citizens' who understand the connections between biomedicine, the wider social world, and the political economy of health" (Robins 2006: 312, 315). With TAC always as the case study, we lost opportunities for seeing empowered citizens in other contexts as well, along with different but equally radical transformations. While I too venerate the successes of TAC and wish for a stronger civil society in Mozambique, I do not think the two countries, or the groups that arose there, are all that comparable.

This book, unfortunately, has primarily been about dysfunction—among patients, in their communities, and in the overarching mechanisms of governance encompassing them. In the posttreatment era, protests and demands have done little to move the therapeutic needle for activists in Mozambique. It may even be fair to say that treatment access in Mozambique would have progressed about as well without the AIDS associations as with them, according to the state of the science and recommendations of health care and development professionals. What we are facing, then, with the Mozambique situation is a set of lost opportunities, underscored by a model of AIDS activism that was superficially supported by the government, financially propped up by NGOs, and ultimately unsustainable. It had room for improvement but never very good guidance.

It is particularly striking how AIDS associations appeared simultaneously threatening to the state (enough to be targeted for registration and standardization) but still inaccessible to the majority of patients in need of a supportive community (inculcated into the world of development projects). Making this possible was an impoverished view of activism—even to the point of using the word *activista* (or activist) to designate paid, salaried positions—and the stunted development of AIDS associations due to conflating the concepts of altruism and production. Participants had to be supportive of one another but still had to compete for funding, limited jobs, and project-related success.

The question I asked in the beginning was the following: what is the role of HIV/AIDS activism and advocacy in the lives of patients in northern Mozambique? The short answer is that it does not transform them into biological citizens. The long answer is only slightly more complicated—AIDS activism, largely writ, allows *some* people to act like biological citizens and then to push their own advantages as far as they can. It serves as a complex set of guidelines for a lucky or ambitious few to wrest power and subsequently benefit disproportionately from those without the means, skills, or desire to participate. AIDS activism becomes yet another type of "governmentality" (Foucault 2010; Lemke 2001; Burchell 1993)—the imposition of certain morals, values, and modes of conduct upon entire groups of people without their obvious and active consent.

There is an important difference, however, in this kind of governmentality because it is not evidently neoliberal in nature. It is, rather, underwritten by biosociality, by the expectation that persons sharing an illness condition are bound by it, and so must or should act together in retaliation or other ways viewed (by outsiders) as essential to offsetting its effects. AIDS activism is, to coin a phrase, a kind of "biosocial governmentality" that is just as capable of shaping mood and desire as any other art of governance, able to strip away diversity in alternative modes of thought and impose itself on future configurations and outcomes.

I have tried here to be faithful to the ethnographic data. In chapter 3, I described intragroup dynamics, dysfunctional meetings and trainings, and the almost oppressive atmosphere of "institutional isomorphism" and "civil society existentialism" in Pemba City. Opportunities related to AIDS activism formed another way for people to *mafiar*—to cheat and to lie—in competition with their friends and neighbors. In chapter 4, I mentioned the basic challenges faced by AIDS activists, NGOs, and home-based care workers in the region. In the "subuniverse" of Cabo Delgado Province poor basic health education, biomedical skepticism, and alcoholism threatened the success of HIV treatment projects. Even in a context of international support for HIV patient groups, still missing were examples of successful support groups for the most common sufferers and victims of the virus.

In chapter 5, failed protests against day hospital closures revealed the futility of rights-based demands and the fractured foundation of the nation's activist community. The presumptions of political process theorists, that engaging in politics was the best way forward for patient groups, were undermined by "slacktivism," which permitted the manipulation of the group by those most interested in being seen and heard in the hope of commerce and employment. Throughout these accounts, what I attempt to make clear is that the needs of HIV-positive people were both basic and prolific, but the Mozambican government was not in a position to adequately respond. State recognition and involvement sparked even more complications. Interdependence with the government and its partners, their passions and politics, compromised the assertiveness and functionality of patient groups. Failed managerial competence filtered down to the level of the group, empowering all the wrong people. Nobody was really in control or ultimately responsible. This was, essentially, a dystopia.

This outcome stands in contrast to the conclusion of prior researchers who studied people with HIV, which zeroed in on the successes and upward trajectory of some patient groups. In Burkina Faso, for example, Nguyen (2007) viewed these groups as effective tools for people living with HIV, even if disruptive to other development work. Noting that levels of high treatment adherence marked an achievement, he introduced "therapeutic citizenship" as a new and unique category of biological citizenship. This pointed to illness claims as a successful bargaining chip for resources in impoverished contexts, much more useful than claims based on poverty, injustice, or structural violence (143).

Robins's (2006) experience with TAC translated into descriptions of people with HIV undergoing powerful identity transformations, from intense states of "near death" to "new life" (313). TAC meetings, and the positive lifestyle associated with group participation, manifested as rites of passage, creating families of fictive kin and leading to stronger, different stages of life. The HIV support group, in these examples, was a source of help or inspiration, allowing people to become "new" selves and "therapeutic citizens," thus freeing them from many aspects of worry and neglect.

In my own research, for a few members, the group did lead to adherence, friendships, and liberation from stigma or anxiety, but for others, it remained a cognitively empty and meaningless space. For some, it intensified distress and fostered jealousy (what Kalofonos [2008] refers to as "biosociopathy"). Such findings resonate strongly with the work of Bähre (2007), who notes that solidarity groups (in this case, for microfinance in Cape Town) do not always result in extensive and unifying bonds of comradeship, especially when explicitly targeted by development work or institutions. According to him, ambivalent relations within groups, and the difficulties of participation and inclusion, must be brought to light if improvements are to be made and hardships lifted. Similarly, Patterson (2016) notes that HIV support groups can be highly unstable. People with HIV in urban Zambia continuously negotiated subjectivity in relation to kinship, their role as clients, and access to resources, leaving them indifferent to political discourse and talk of inclusion, what she dubs "therapeutic pacifism." Taken together, these more recent studies indicate that biosociality, and what it produces in different contexts, unravels or is not very predictable.

Marsland's work in rural Tanzania (2012) questions if a seropositive status, or a life dependent on ART, is at all sufficient for biosocial groups to even develop. *Huruma*, one of the HIV support groups she studied, had difficulty recruiting members out of fear their status would become known. This is undoubtedly a challenge in rural areas, as I noted in chapter 4, where there seems to be much less to gain from disclosing one's status in close-knit communities. Biosociality, Marsland mentions, is present as people help one another adhere to medication and stay healthy, but this is not a result of newly formed HIV patient groups. The biosocial paths that she charted were laid down along "already existing networks of family and neighbors" (473). She suggests the most interesting forms of biosociality are the least obvious, composed of isolated individuals who do not wish to disclose their status and circles of friends not registered as official or formal groups. These point to the existence of a "hidden collective" (474) not as readily studied as biological citizenship but still important in anthropological understandings of biosociality. If biosociality does not progress or move toward biological citizenship, then privileging or highlighting AIDS activism may block other, legitimate biosocial pathways.

One way around this might be to talk less about citizenship and more about different biosocialities. In that line of thought, what we are dealing with, potentially, are at least two competing "types" of biosocialities—one dominant, the other not. We have, in the dominant type, the concept of the new self, of re-creation, of the group and its members hyperinvolved in facets of lobbying, raising funds, promoting research, or educating the masses. They proudly serve as living, breathing examples of an escape from victimhood. This is the biosociality of the benevolent social actor, whose participation in articulatory politics, even at minimum levels, serves to redefine perceptions about him, her, or the group in ways intended to build it up from the outside in.

We have, second. and in the nondominant biosociality, the concept of taking back a lost life, of picking up where one left off, of not necessarily reaching for something new but regaining something lost. These seek to reinsert themselves back into society without drawing special attention or making specific demands upon it. This is the biosociality of domestic security, encouraging participation with the group as it is centered on obtaining composure and esteem following a major life disruption. The embrace of either biosociality—the dominant or the nondominant type—is subject to personal preference but also to marketing techniques, the availability of various strains of thought, and the deployment of terms, images, and concepts that brush up against and become tangible in the hearts and minds of the populace. Biological citizenship may just be an "aggressive" form of biosociality, more available to those who have chosen (or been conferred with) its dominant type.

The challenge for the HIV patient group, and the anthropologist who studies it, is to acknowledge that various or competing biosocialities are relevant and that much work remains to be done regarding this unmapped typology. If this does not happen, the threat to be faced is that of biological citizenship as a civilizing mission—the implication that people are "better off" that way. Like the Portuguese or the British in colonial southern Africa, who claimed projects of social uplift and integration, this threat masquerades as a promise of dissipating ignorance, of drawing marginalized persons into a global economy, and of a promised future world of success or opportunity. Giving in to this threat, in less-developed nations, the prototype of the AIDS activist parallels that of the freed slave or the noble savage, not so much in content as in poise, offered up as a literary stock character to which we can point and reference without much thought or wasted space in an article or term paper.

But a high price is attached to the use of tropes, paid in myopic snippets rather than kernels of truth and in the whittling down of activists such that they are no longer determinants of themselves. An obsession with spectacle has created a taste for activism and its novelties, pushing some concerns into public life. Demands that get met are mostly logistical, such as the distance from home to clinic, the distribution of material resources, or numbers of bodies on treatment. Demands that get ignored or even ridiculed are deeper and more far-reaching, such as self-mastery, moral inventories, and the minimization of harmful behaviors.

To truly be countercultural, AIDS activism cannot embrace the same currency and language of the very institutions it claims to attack. Power, recognition, influence, even formal employment, these are not lofty goals for the group, but neither are they sufficient means to an end or always worthwhile endeavors. The common support group is unable to accomplish the socially and economically desirable objectives that should be within its own reach. Channeled, funded, and forced to operate within externally imposed strictures and limits, we find the topic at a dead end, in the throes of dissolution. By allowing biological citizenship to become the goal of biosociality, therapy is no longer truly the point, and we find ourselves unable to differentiate between capital and hope, between producing a "worthy" illness (Berliner and Kenworthy 2017) or engaging vulnerable people on their own terms. Activism as we know it seems to have gone this route: it has been expendable, temporary, a mere puff of wind, likewise for many HIV patient groups in the region.

CARIDADE'S FINAL ELECTION

"Somos a resistência [we are the resistance]," said Falume, sitting on my veranda in Bairro Eduardo Mondlane the night before Caridade's third and what would turn out to be final *assembleia* (election). He was referring to a faction within Caridade that intended to see Luisa lose her upcoming run for the presidency. This time, the third election for the association, Antonio's term limits had maxed out, so somebody new would be taking the reins for the first time. Together with Fevereiro (the presidential candidate other than Luisa), Carlitos (my research assistant, running for Fevereiro's former position of treasurer), and a new member of Caridade, Fevereiro's drunken neighbor (who would soon be installed as an activist in the group, even though he had never taken an HIV test), we were doing what men do in the evening with extra available foreign funding—drinking beers.

The foreign funding came from my Fulbright award money, of which I had some remaining as the weeks wound down prior to my departure from the country and back to East Lansing, Michigan. Another activist, Hamisi, a member of both Caridade and Bem Vindo, had just joined us, coming from the Medicos del Mundo compound farther up the beach and toward town. He was complaining about having to end a recent sexual tryst with an Italian expatriate because "our relationship was messed up," he told us. "I left her because I didn't want to be abused by these people. . . . They treat us blacks as if they are colonizers."

But he had other business there as well, that of trying to *organizar alguma coisa* (organize something) to eat and drink from that particular donor for Caridade's elections. In Pemba, this phrase is a classic marker of the *pedido*—an "asking" or a begging. I had been privy to this particular negotiation, which started several days before. The coordinator of Medicos del Mundo approached me during a training they were holding to raise awareness of the virus on the part of local male barbers in the area (who, it was assumed, tended to have rather frank sexual discussions with clients and so were supposedly suitable outlets for handing out condoms). Toni, the Spanish coordinator, told me he was very saddened by Caridade's list of requested items for the election, which included thirty-seven chickens, twenty cases of beer, twenty kilograms of maize meal and rice, and host of other goods that he deemed to be excessive or inappropriate for a six-hour meeting.

It occurred to me that he wasn't aware of exactly how these kinds of negotiations work. People and groups, especially Caridade, try to get all that they can from donors. This is because they have no idea when they will have another legitimate opportunity to ask for things but also because if you start out big, then the final take is likely to be better than if you start out small. It's always a process, these kinds of negotiations, not much different from any other kind of business deal, just like haggling in a market over tomatoes or bananas or naming the price to be paid to a day laborer. Each side tries to do the best for themselves that they can. Hamisi, aside from having ditched his relatively new foreign lover, had also just secured what Caridade needed to feed the sixty or so members it had on election day—most of the food but none of the beer.

Just then, Luisa rang Fevereiro on his cellular phone. He answered and greeted her, then activated the speakerphone, giving us the signal to be quiet. "We have to punish Teresa," said Luisa.

"And why is that?" Fevereiro replied, looking both amused and perplexed. Teresa was one of those activists who worked in programs for both Caridade and Bem Vindo, a long-standing member of both associations, whose entire family and neighborhood knew her positive status and her work in HIV education and home-based care. She got a hefty month's salary from her involvement with both groups.

"She didn't turn in her report last month," Luisa continued, "I'm going to cut one month's salary from her." At this, Carlitos looked at me and smiled sadly. We both knew that Luisa's intention was to take that money for herself, and if necessary, share it with Fevereiro to get him on her side in any ensuing debate with Teresa as a result of losing the money.

"Sister," said Fevereiro, "I have that report. It's on my desk. Teresa brought it to me last week."

"No, but that's too late," Luisa replied, "she always does that, and one day it's going to make us lose funding." Fevereiro wrapped up the conversation off speakerphone, telling Luisa that he would come and discuss it with her the next day. The group briefly discussed this exchange. These days, Luisa never came to the office anymore but instead just stayed at home, making demands to other Caridade leaders over the phone. If that weren't the case, she would have seen Teresa's report and wouldn't even have broached this subject with Fevereiro. For his part, Fevereiro asked me if I had any *agua de papa* (daddy's drink) in the fridge because he knew I often kept whiskey in there. I handed him the bottle.

In the weeks leading up to Caridade's third election, almost all work around the office stopped. However, circulating among the homes of members and activists, it became clear that the energy normally devoted to that was being put into private meetings and low-level bribery. The two running for president, Luisa and Fevereiro, both had "their people." Loyalty to either depended mostly on which one had conferred activist status and salary to a particular person, and in terms of that, Luisa clearly had the majority. Her efforts at campaigning centered on the art of the strategic phone call, coupled with entertaining members she considered to be capable of influencing others by inviting them to her home for dinner or drinks. Fevereiro's approach was much more laissez-faire. He allowed others to campaign on his behalf. Because he was more often present at the office, making him more accessible and approachable, and because he was not as high profile as Luisa, who did talks on the radio and headed up city-wide meetings, people considered Fevereiro a safe and nonpolitical alternative.

Many feared that Luisa would take the association over completely if she won, by continuing to appoint young, HIV-negative friends to paid positions. The older, founding members of Caridade saw Luisa as an upstart, and were likely to vote for Fevereiro because he was also a founder. Caridade's policy was that the presidential candidate to receive the second most votes would become vice-president. A third candidate, Zaida, was a relative unknown. Most knew that she ran at the request of Luisa, who was hoping to split the votes so that hers added up to more than Fevereiro's.

The candidates for the other positions—secretary, treasurer, president of the assembly, and *porta-voz* (messenger)—were a mix of activists who regularly showed up around the office. Some of these were actively buying votes from members in the form of drinks purchased from barracas across the street or giving small amounts of cash to select people. One day, after closing up his office, the accountant Bakari handed me 300 Mozambican meticais (about U.S.$12), and I wasn't even a voting member of the association. He just smiled and pointed discretely to Falume, who was running again for president of the assembly but had his back turned and didn't notice the exchange. There was an obvious rise in the number of private walks that people took together leading up to the elections, where strategies and discussions could be had in secret, away from prying eyes and curious ears, and under the pretense of just catching up.

Elected Caridade leaders served five-year terms, were guaranteed a salary (in meticais) that whole time, and have the final say in the lives of activists. They approved their reports, their vacation requests, and collectively represented all the supervisorial duties common to any other business, company, or organization. Therefore, there was strong competition to get elected to these positions: jobs of any nature in Pemba City were highly sought after. Unfortunately, Caridade leaders depended on the organizations that financed the group, which included at that time Action Aid, FOCADE, RENSIDA, MONASO, and the Núcleo. When any of those donors sneezed, Caridade caught the cold. This was the group's eventual fate—almost complete defunding.

The election went off without a hitch. Action Aid paid for the supplies and renting the room at the Red Cross, and there was enough food and soda for everybody. Prior to each round of voting, the candidates were permitted to give a brief speech, summarizing the reason for their interest, their accomplishments, what skills they brought to the table, and how the association would benefit from their service. Many, including Carlitos, my research assistant, employed the language of human rights and the need to fight for better services and more projects. Others stressed their long-standing loyalty to Caridade, having not defected to join or found other AIDS associations. Still others emphasized their educational credentials, their capacity to write proposals and apply and secure funding.

Those who had spoken so loudly and boldly in small group settings leading up to the election seemed tamed and even intimidated in the rather formal atmosphere of the large room in which we sat, sixty to seventy Caridade members, ready to write down someone's name and decide their future. Fevereiro won the presidency, and Luisa became vice-president for the second time. Hamisi became secretary, Carlitos the treasurer, and Falume continued as president of the assembly. Antonio, my first contact with the association, its founder, and two-term president, didn't show up to vote. I would only see him again one time before his death in 2013, the result, so I was told, of too much drinking. He left behind a widow and two children.

Over the next few weeks, my last bit of time with the association, Caridade worked as if powered by a million horses. However, the reason for this was not the regime change, it was fear. The association in the nearby town of Nampula had lost its contract with UNICEF through RENSIDA—the primary-school HIV awareness project that also provided support to orphans and vulnerable children. External monitoring of the group's efforts revealed certain irregularities that didn't add up to a justifiable budge, and the program was cut. The very thought of this happening to Caridade was terrifying to everybody.

The UNICEF contract made up the bread and butter, the majority of funds, for Caridade, excepting the Action Aid money that paid for the office and some occasional community programs in Pemba City. Loss of the UNICEF project would also mean the loss of Caridade's presence in the rest of Cabo Delgado Province. What all this meant is that Caridade had to get its records and its story straight about the UNICEF project in multiple sites. Receipts had to be obtained for purchases and, if that wasn't possible, forged and then re-signed by the appropriate people. Reported calendar dates of implementation had to be correct and correspond to those on submitted progress reports. Evaluations of trainings and projects had to be collected and organized and appear legitimate. Goods distributed and services rendered had to be well documented. Transportation for project oversight had to be justified. All this presented a huge conceptual task to the association because of the many corners cut in the recent past.

There were times, for example, that trips to the provinces simply didn't happen. Caridade supervisors were supposed to make regularly scheduled visits to places like Balama, Montepuez, Chiure, Meluco, and Muidumbe, all within the province but requiring overnight trips at least. There were instances when transportation broke down or somebody got sick, and the visit was canceled. Trainings were supposed to be conducted with new activists or in schools with the beneficiaries. Some of these were cut short. Others had been compromised by Caridade's partner on the project, Pemba's Ministry of Education, which sometimes added new people to the project and tried to insert its own activists into Caridade's activities, leading to shorter or less-effective efforts because funding didn't stretch as far. Surprisingly, though, approval for another three-year period was granted (after my departure) in early 2010 for Caridade to continue administering the UNICEF project, which was ultimately cut nationwide in 2012. That was the time when everything else began to fizzle out for the group as well.

By 2015, Caridade still had a rented office, but the door remained mostly shut. Plans to buy land and build a new office to be owned by the group had been abandoned. From 2012 to 2015, the association got USAID funding, through a well-known contractor, for initiatives to help support civil society. That grant—according to Carlitos, who was no longer participating—paid salaries for five "experts" and three "activists," expecting all other association members to volunteer their time. This effectively reduced Caridade's numbers to eight people and because Luisa had somehow become the sole administrator of that project, they were all her friends and family. Since then, other Caridade leaders have turned to different kinds of business in order to support themselves, and the only AIDS association that continues to function, in 2017, is the one funded by PEPFAR through the Elizabeth Glazer Pediatric AIDS Foundation—Bem Vindo—whose members are mostly not HIV positive. The other HIV support groups in the city and surrounding municipalities have completely folded.

WHERE NOW ARE THE BIOLOGICAL CITIZENS?

Despite the demise of Caridade, and many other HIV support groups and associations, lip service is still paid to groups like these even as they are disappearing, and HIV-specific programming and clinics have been shut down. A kind of political doublespeak persists at the level of those with the most decision-making power that tends to drown out the voices of those to whom they claim to cater. UNAIDS places Mozambique into a category of countries "with generalized epidemics, low antiretroviral therapy coverage and high gaps in treatment access" (UNAIDS 2012: 39). Here, we were told, "special efforts are required to maintain and accelerate scale-up in these countries" (39).

Claiming to recognize an unfinished agenda associated with full ART coverage, the document *Treatment 2015* (UNAIDS 2012) called on civil society to do exactly what they were doing before, to be more engaged with advocacy and accountability, service delivery, and community mobilization. People with HIV were called on to help health service facilities identify factors contributing to slow treatment uptake and program dropout (36). Yet what actually happened was the opposite of all these proscriptions. Compared to just a few years ago, in Mozambique, there are no special efforts, except health systems strengthening and performance-based financing, aimed at the level of bureaucracy and government contracting. As opposed to institutions, the manner in which communities of people with HIV were able to persist together in Mozambique—through the AIDS association—was decimated from both the inside and out.

While UNAIDS goes on to talk about the need for the "widest array of partners" including community-based organizations and people living with HIV, particularly in order to generate demand for treatment, inform strategy development, and support service delivery (2012: 36), these groups have been cut off from the funding pipeline through what appears to be a well-concerted effort. Organizations like Medicos del Mundo, the Clinton Foundation, and MSF—the groups that funded and worked most closely with AIDS associations—have been told to move on to addressing the entire patient population. For the most part, they have complied. Yet for some reason, the large, multinational programs and institutions like UNAIDS and PEPFAR continue their work on HIV and AIDS only. The juxtaposition is circumspect in its disregard for average patients but fits well into the concept of a "planned shrinkage" (Wallace 1990: 427), the "landscape of despair" (Dear and Wolch 1987) that might, with different sources of thought and input, have been avoided.

Official reports and mainstream literature acknowledge the fact that the AIDS activist, as biological citizen, is less and less able to harbor ill will against the system. Programs and projects are able to point to the AIDS activist as included in their plans. This corresponds strongly to the viability of productive logic, of the dangers imposed when constitutive labor is mistaken for patient advocacy. It might be that the government and its partners wanted to try their hands at patient identity formation. This would be useful for later tearing it apart but still reaping the rewards. The Mozambican AIDS associations provided that sort of platform, where there was nothing to lose. From an investor's perspective, their long-term sustainability meant nothing. Working expediently at the level of their desires, offering jobs and salaries and promotions, had a sublimely negative effect on the group's concepts of fairness and ethics. It had an equally opposite effect on its aggregate potentiality, a safe bet that the proliferation of AIDS associations would yield a positive return on investments and eventual surplus value.

HIV patient groups—and day hospitals as well—have been excellent sites for venture capital, testing receptivity before ramping up treatment. Indications of success in smaller settings pointed to greater successes in other places and, with bodies previously inaccessible but no longer unreachable, the rest of the population. The state, inserting itself into activism and by later silently withdrawing, was able to leave it worse off than if it had never even been involved. AIDS activism, by toying with the state, encountered very different results. With its membership base sullied from competition and irredeemable from the conflict and slander, the limits of solidarity were tested and did not hold up. The presupposed alliance between those sharing the same predicament or illness broke down, an outcome suggesting that biosociality and activism do not always see eye-to-eye and do not peacefully coexist.

This ill-founded relationship came to fruition with the decentralization of day hospitals, which was likewise the decentralization of an HIV-positive patient consciousness. The failure here of AIDS activism was not in its inability to silence its critics or speak out but in its murky capacity for justifying itself through evidence. Had patient-activists observed that their existence was contingent on production and not really on human rights, then the benefits of nondominant forms of biosociality, and the imperative for domestic security over benevolent social action, may have assumed a position of authority. In a world that kowtows more to efficiency than ideals, "movements" besides only social ones carry and disseminate their own messages. The "evidence-based policy movement" (Sundell and Wärngård 2013: 12) permitted Garrido to ignore the gap between his decision and prevailing activist sentiments. Regardless of the fact that sufficient time and effort had not been invested to distill exactly how these wide-scale changes might be felt in every context, universal patient rights overtook AIDS activism on the international list of key issues. To stay on the side of management processes, politicians respond better to talking points than to populist demands.

The loss of external support would have been less impactful had HIV-positive patients been seeking benefits from their collective involvement other than material resources. Were groups more effectively bent on the prevention of disease relapse among their own members and the dissemination of illness-coping or livelihood strategies exclusive from external programs, then the capacity for AIDS activism to drive health data and outcomes in its own right would have been better parsed. Up against "the market" as a site for doing things quickly and efficiently, treatment as a form of self-improvement is easily withdrawn or transferred out of the group. The project plan, as well, is revealed as a technique simply on loan.

The eventual unwillingness to allocate any power to AIDS activism had everything to do with a lack of competing proofs in defense of what the group was always better equipped for than the state. Destigmatizing the virus at the community level, highlighting the scale of the pandemic in the realm of the social, the circulation of social capital, and inculcation into moral economies are items and tasks less easy to measure than most others, but they are more than mere fillers in the lives of the afflicted. We are at a point where logical demonstrations are preferable to demonstrations in the street.

Without rosters, leaders, project money, or talking to the press, Alcoholics Anonymous is the most successful support group model in the world. Reconciling people with life as a safe place, replete with practical advice and social support, these groups do not furnish members with jobs, salaries, or housing. They accept no outside funds nor do they rely on medical professionals and experts for guidance. Yet they proliferate internationally and each meeting differs according to speakers and content. "Sponsors" care for new members and lead them through standard steps that liberate people from harmful thinking and negative behavior. Rather than seeking out formal programs, formal programs seek out the group, sending sick people to the community for therapy that clinicians can't provide. Aspects of apprenticeship, addressing the existential vacuum, and exploration of meaning and sacrifice—these are viable goals for the group but less so for the state and still measurable in number of lives saved (Frankl 2006). Social realism is social justice (Archer 1995), and the promotion of dignity is as practical of a concern as any other (Rosen 2012). In the hyperpoliticized world of HIV care, there increasingly seems to be no place for such a model.

There is something to be said, then, for the absence of gatekeepers. It may increase emotional commitment and obligation and decrease the tension between institutional formation and community loyalty. It may better enable the stabilization of self-consciousness and the transfer of experiential knowledge and carve out space for appeals that differ from those linked mostly to representation and entitlement. There may be many points of dissonance between "expert" activists and self-advocates, which remain obscured out of fear they might upset normality. But this normality is the result of a "looping effect" (Hacking 2000), where activism becomes self-referential and ceases to align outside of its own expectations. There were different sorts of problems, of affect and mood, difficult to broach in Mozambican AIDS associations at the very outset. Equally accessible and utilized as the language of solidarity is that of disappointment, exclusion, and lost opportunity that indicates politics is no longer fertile ground. AIDS activism is haunted by this lack of foundational emotional and even discursive work. Protests against it have taken the form of apathy, disinterest, and detachment.

What we have, then, are scores of homeless biological citizens who set their sights on the wrong kind of citizenship. Striving and inspired to become citizens of the transnational, but less motivated as citizens of the local, perceived opportunities for self-enrichment combined with poor guidance and oversight led to internal group sabotage and professional inefficacy. Activism serves as a distraction and insufficient moral ground for group cohesion. The blending together of projects both public and private is like serving two masters, enabling personal agendas to overtake the common good. By now work on the self, at the level of greed or the slaking of similar unhealthy thirsts, is more than necessary, it's required. The topic of responsibilization, confessional technologies, and testimonials should be revisited. Bereft of lay psychology, the group is more likely to become a tool for the elite than a forum for the disadvantaged.

To follow a motto or mantra would have been a good start. The names of AIDS associations encapsulate the mission. *Caridade* refers to unconditional love. *Bem Vindo* means welcome. *Nashukuru* is thankfulness. *Ajuda à Próxima* is help your neighbor. *Esperanca da Vida* is hope of life. These concepts are not foreign but fail to direct action so long as they remain uninspired. While making connections between politics, projects, and patient groups is not always and everywhere wrong, the approach has mostly been speculative. "Humans existence is always oriented toward the future," writes sociologist (and social constructivist) Peter Berger (1970: 61). In other words, we exist by constantly extending our being into the future, both in our consciousness and in our activity. Put differently, we realize ourselves in projects. An essential dimension of this "futurity" of humanity is hope. It is through hope that we overcome the difficulties of any given here and now.

Where the AIDS associations failed was in the project of hope. Every stolen goat, every misspent dollar, every missed chance for a meeting not just about resources and expenses were slaps in the face of the ordinary HIV-positive patient and his or her hopes and dreams. The groups in Cabo Delgado would have been better off without such projects. Abuse of the project is the doorway to abuse of the group. It is apparent to everybody; the secrets are not easily hidden. This is how AIDS associations failed to impact the society around them, robbing their own future, inviting their takeover by the outspoken, the clever, and the corrupt.

The capitalist rationality fueling the expansion of government into the lives and minds of people has no problem with elements of social conflict. Protests, civil society disruptions, claims made against the state provide less opportunity for social advancement than at first it seems. The "opportunity" of a struggle, even when it results in an apparent accumulation of goods (or access to treatment), signals also the group's affability at being worked on, defined, and shaped in a manner it might not expect. Aspiring to universality, the global village, or the transnational nature of HIV/AIDS patienthood lends itself well to domination by others. Not only is it easy to challenge in terms of practice, but its application requires an attack on diversity, leading to a platform on which all can agree, usually evoking one or another version of *the consumer*.

Millikan (1987) posits the consumer as a hungry frog, darting out its tongue to consume any material appropriate in size that moves past its retinas. Unsure of its content—it could be poisonous—we can look to the frog to see if it was appropriate or not. As the food moves downstream, we can also gauge how well it benefits the creatures in different environs. Are the creatures altered, sickly, or more energetic? Does the content have the same effects as it moves further from its source? The folding of patient groups at my research sites, and subsequent lack of replacements, suggest the content did not satiate. Perhaps it was inappropriate; perhaps it satisfied minimally, at the level only of primary desire, of instant gratification.

But it is not wrong to want. MacIntyre offers the concept of enlightened self-interest as not at all incompatible with seeking "the good life" (1999: 13), but power, money, and influence alone do not further cooperative pursuits. The figure of the AIDS activist, at the forefront of a vanguard of social justice, offers no way out of "the state" versus "the excluded" dilemma (Santos 2005). As this figure draws us more and more into a cycle of participation, it will become less provocative despite its birth in the fire of rights and demands. This biological citizen also offers us no way out of the Foucauldian snares laid out in concepts of governmentality and biopolitical power, perceived as ineliminable life elements and constant disruptions.

Displacing (neo)liberalism—as a hindrance to civil society, as a constraint on freedom or the autonomy of the group—rests on the practices, rationality, and morality of "plain persons" (MacIntyre 1999: 15), those whom Nietzsche (1989) identifies as "the herd." Identities based on biological facts take shape in ways not nearly as unruly as previously thought. The consequences are really rather predictable. Investors want consumers and the state wants participants. Both are happy to intervene because it legitimizes their presence, spurring business and politics onward.

Normalcy for the group, and the establishment of effective support networks, was a persistent design flaw for AIDS activism in southern Africa. Attempts to correct it unsurprisingly corresponded to preexisting patterns, the same kinds that often establish themselves after the discovery of an illness, its treatment, and related biosociality. This hasn't occurred ad hoc but through highlights of heroism, utopias, and exemplary case studies, simultaneously indicative both of activism's monopoly on public symbols and their spoliative effects. The failure to communicate worry, distress, fear, frustration, and anxiety eclipses paths for moderation and correction. Bad work and poor performance do not constitute research material to be discarded, as often thought, and should instead be integrated into the construction of narratives to help us assess the past and plan for the future.

But confusion continues. We still believe AIDS activism is more about medicine and complaints than quality of life. The "fourth wave" of AIDS activism (Smith 2013) is attributed once again to patients demanding treatment, this time for preexposure prophylaxis, treatment as prevention, and forced taxes on Wall Street to fund progressive causes. Such concerns stand in for and replace the need to rethink relations between governance, society, and chronic patienthood. Locked in this cycle, it is unlikely for biosociality to positively develop much further. Treatment is for people, not people for treatment, but emerging only for crises or in apparent states of disrepair, HIV/AIDS civil society and AIDS activism presents itself as destined, if not prepackaged, mostly for consumerism and scandal. We find ourselves still waiting on a satisfactory defense of the local, the average, the common, and the humble.

NOTES

INTRODUCTION

1. I worked with eight different AIDS associations in Cabo Delgado Province. Names of associations have been changed to protect their identity. Names of informants, likewise, have been changed for purposes of confidentiality.
2. See http://hdr.undp.org/en/countries/profiles/MOZ for these statistics.
3. The global Multidimensional Poverty Index (MPI) is a composite indicator that assesses the intensity of poverty at the individual level. Used by the U.N. and released annually, it replaces the Human Poverty Index, which measured health, education, and living standards. The MPI uses each of these but expands them to encompass the following: child mortality, nutrition, years of schooling, school attendance, cooking fuel, toilet, water, electricity, floor, and assets (such as property and household items). An MPI of 70 percent means that in Mozambique more than two-thirds of residents are "MPI poor," or deprived in at least one-third of these indicators (statistically weighted).

CHAPTER 1   STUDYING HIV AND HIV-POSITIVE PERSONS

1. HIV was first called the human T-cell leukemia virus and later the human T-cell lymphotropic virus when first uncovered through oncology investigations at the United States National Cancer Institute (NCI) in 1980. It was identified independently in France three years later as the lymphadenopathy associated virus (Lapierre 1990). As the viral hypothesis was further explored and elaborated, it was later termed the AIDS-related virus (Shilts 1987), eventually characterized as an infectious disease and renamed the human immunodeficiency virus, or HIV (Piel 1988).
2. Responding to activist demands, the CDC expanded the definition of AIDS in 1993 to include not just deaths but CD4 T-cell counts, pulmonary tuberculosis, recurrent pneumonia, and invasive cervical cancer. Chapter 2 of Alexis Shotwell's book *Against Purity* (2016) tracks this transition very well.
3. The incorporation of HIV testing in population-based surveys resulted in decreasing estimates of global burden around 2006 (UNAIDS 2006). Random testing and the inclusion of men complemented antenatal clinic surveillance, leading to a more accurate model and lower official numbers in most countries.
4. While the production, circulation, use, and evaluation of empirical scientific "evidence" has played a central role in activists' engagement with AIDS science, it need not be so in the case of support groups. As Colvin (2014) points out, controversies over new treatment and prevention approaches can either mobilize or create friction in activist circles. Debates raging regarding B+, microbicides, male circumcision, treatment as prevention, preexposure prophylaxis (PrEP), test-and-treat, provider-initiated testing, managed ART, and the timing of treatment for TB/HIV coinfection underscore the need for support groups to remain focused on peer counseling and not become embroiled in the arguments of scientists, lab technicians, and technocrats.

5. For an excellent on-screen depiction of this phenomenon, see *Dallas Buyer's Club* (Vallée 2013).

6. I refer here to the Community ART Support Groups (CASGs) pioneered in Tete by MSF and taken up nationally by the Ministry of Health. The next solid wave of research on HIV-positive persons might take into account these smaller (four- to six-person) groups. Strictly oriented toward pill-taking, by decree, an interesting next Mozambican project would explore their sociopolitical value and potential for community uplift and identity formation (Jobarteh et al. 2016).

7. Now called SERVE Zambia Foundation, Pastor Andrew Kayekesi founded this community-based organization before moving on to serve as mayor of Luanshya.

CHAPTER 2   "MOVEMENTS" OF THE PAST

1. For the most recent definitive ethnography on Mueda and Makonde people, see Kupilikula (West 2005) and its fascinating depictions of early Frelimo life in the bush.

2. The Shirazi people are a Swahili-speaking ethnic group of Persian or Iranian origin whose commercial and economic livelihood was mercantile and seafaring in nature. Their extensive and long history in East Africa, dating back to the tenth century, is associated with gold and the slave trade, the spread of Sufi Islam, highly interconnected clanships, and palatial home bases, which included Kilwa in Kenya, Unguja and Pemba (Zanzibar) in Tanzania, various other sultanates (including Angoche in Mozambique), and parts of the Comoros Islands (Mutiua 2014; Bonate 2015).

3. The Agreement on Trade-Related Aspects of Intellectual Property Rights (TRIPS) is an international legal agreement between all member nations of the World Trade Organization (WTO). It imposes minimum standards for many forms of intellectual property (IP), including but not limited to pharmaceutical patents. Due to its focus on copyrights and trademarks, critics of TRIPS understood the following threats to drug access in developing nations: increased (corporate) patent protection leading to higher drug prices; negative effects on local manufacturing capacity, removing sources of generic medications; and inadequate encouragement of research and development for drugs with low profit potential (especially for diseases like tuberculosis and malaria). The Doha Declaration was issued as an amendment to TRIPS, viewed as relaxing limitations in poorer countries. Doha emphasized that TRIPS should not prevent governments from protecting public health and that access to medicines for all was a guarantee, particularly if member states declared a public health emergency. Seen as necessary for striking a balance between encouraging innovation and the use of existing creations, TRIPS brought debates over drug access to the forefront, as corporations, governments, and special interest groups all sought protection from the agreement and modifications to its language, timelines, and effects in various settings ('t Hoen 2002).

CHAPTER 4   CHALLENGES TO HIV/AIDS ACTIVISM IN THE "SUBUNIVERSE" OF CABO DELGADO

1. This phrase builds on the work of Berger and Luckmann (1967), who talk about "the man in the street" and the need for the social scientist to differentiate between the knowledge-realities of philosophers and that of the general public. Since their phrase was not gender neutral, I have chosen to revise it, although I do not otherwise seek to modify or detract from the initial application of the concept. It permits the inclusion of local beliefs and the fact that we can take them seriously, even if they appear wrong to science and related brands of authority:

"specific agglomerations of 'reality' and 'knowledge' pertain to specific social contexts, and these relationships will have to be included in an adequate sociological analysis of these contexts" (2).

2. Use of the word "tribe" connotes a conceptual conundrum in anthropology (Mafeje 1976). I do not imply tacit approval of Africa's colonial past but seek instead to apprehend bounded notions of identity and vernacular that escape efficient description. Applied also today to Wall Street bankers (Ho 2009) and laboratory scientists (Spencer and Walby 2013), tribalism sparks discussion too weighty to be adequately addressed here.

3. This statement is partly true. Mozambique's first AIDS case was diagnosed in 1986 in Pemba. However, it was a black Haitian American man, not a white man (Matsinhe 2008: 36).

4. See Afzal et al. (2015) for a medically-based discussion of peripheral neuropathy in advanced HIV disease, which tends to begin with lower-extremity weakness, numbness, and tingling sensations that eventually spread throughout the body.

CHAPTER 5   THE (DIS)INTEGRATION OF THE DAY HOSPITALS

1. Matsinhe mentions the intense negotiations that occurred over the creation of other specialty AIDS projects—like the National AIDS Council and the implementation of AIDS-only strategic action plans (PEN I, II, and III; 2008: 55–73). Day hospitals, likewise, may have been considered unwieldy.

2. WHO guidelines around eligibility criteria began to change in Mozambique in 2009, the same year of the HDD closures. Changes were implemented to raise the CD4 count from ≤200 cells/mm to 350, expanding the eligible population and making coverage appear lower (worse). Estimates in Spectrum, the software used to model ART coverage data, were formerly presented in Mozambique's annual reports in two ways. The first way, which is now phased out, used "patients eligible for ART" as the denominator. An example is graphic 3 of MISAU (2015)—with coverage at 56 percent. These data show declining coverage from 2008 to 2012. However, it is not possible to attribute this either to HDD closures or changes in eligibility criteria based on the available information; even total conformity to the CD4 ≤ 350 from one clinic site to another is subject to debate. The second way to model these data uses "HIV-positive persons" as the denominator—showing 13 percent coverage. This method, while decidedly more precise, likewise prohibits distinguishing the impact of the HDD closures on ART coverage during the time period in question.

3. Mr. Mufanequico indirectly highlights an important point here: the word "decentralization" seems counterintuitive and illogical. A better word for the process would have been "centralization," referring to the government takeover and desire to manage the clinics. The next section will clarify the history of the word in Africa, which emerged from a lexicon of available concepts and partly explains why it was chosen. However, it is helpful to keep in mind that state and donor use of the word "decentralization" refers not to decision-making power but to health services. Health care "decentralization" signifies offering services like ART in more clinics as opposed to "central" or limited locations like urban hospitals (or HDDs). Use of the word "integration" in tandem further specifies the intention and trajectory of the change, as HDDs get "integrated" into other clinics from their previous solitary status, allowing treatment services to get pushed out again to government-run clinics (or "decentralized").

4. There were two exceptions to this. The Centro de Saúde do Alto Maé in Maputo (run by MSF) and the day hospital at Maputo's military hospital—both out of the Ministry of Health's reach—continued to function up until 2013.

5. Percentages of women and men fifteen to forty-nine years old who are HIV positive by province, Mozambique, 2009 and 2015.

6. Percentage HIV positive among women and men who were tested, Mozambique, 2009 and 2015.

7. Percentages of women and men fifteen to forty-nine years old who, in response to prompted questions, say that people can reduce the risk of getting HIV by using condoms every time they have sexual intercourse and by having one sex partner who is not infected and has no other partners, Mozambique, 2003 to 2015.

8. Percentages of women and men fifteen to forty-nine years old who know that the consistent use of condoms during sexual intercourse and having just one uninfected partner can reduce the chances of getting HIV, know that a healthy-looking person can have HIV, and reject the two most common local misconceptions about transmission or prevention of HIV (that it can be contracted through mosquito bites or eating with an HIV-positive person), Mozambique, 2003 to 2015.

9. Percentages of women and men fifteen to twenty-four years old who know that the consistent use of condoms during sexual intercourse and having just one uninfected partner can reduce the chances of getting HIV, know that a healthy-looking person can have HIV, and reject the two most common local misconceptions about transmission or prevention of HIV (that it can be contracted through mosquito bites or eating with an HIV-positive person), Mozambique, 2003 to 2015.

10. Percentages of women and men fifteen to forty-nine years old who know that HIV can be transmitted from mother to child by breastfeeding and that the risk of mother-to-child transmission of HIV can be reduced by the mother taking special drugs during pregnancy, Mozambique, 2003 to 2015.

11. The preference for quantitative metrics (Adams 2016) and other enumerative practices (Sangaramoorthy and Benton 2012) is of increasing concern in medical anthropology. "Who benefits from crisis and response?" "What kind of political arrangements unfold?" and "To what extent do old systems of dependence get recreated?" remain open-ended and unanswered questions. Moreover, standards that govern data collection and reporting can reproduce the shared understandings of those in control of resources and funding (Biruk 2012). Trepidation over PBF, emanating as it does from prevailing governing structures, falls along these same lines, related to the imposition of market logics and the molding or shaping of cultural and institutional norms.

12. See the website for ThinkWell Global, http://thinkwell.global/projects/performance-based-financing-for-mozambique/.

13. Affiliated with USAID through the private sector contractor John Snow Inc.

14. Recent anthropological work around the "normalization" of HIV (Philbin 2014; McGrath et al. 2014) recognizes that when depicted as a chronic, manageable illness, challenging realities of living with the virus get downplayed. These include the costs of seeking treatment in contexts of severe poverty and persistent stigma (Mattes 2014) as well as questioning the relationship between treatment literacy and drug efficacy (Niehaus 2014). Just as the dominant clinical narrative—that routine access to care is sufficient for returning to a normal life—does not adequately address the full range of PWA experiences, applied here, normalization suggests that neither does health systems strengthening erase the need either for solidarity among illness sufferers or safe spaces for them to congregate and receive care.

15. Success stories in neighboring countries Swaziland, Zambia, Malawi, and Zimbabwe indicate greater gains than in Mozambique. PEPFAR suggests those countries are

approaching epidemic control, especially in Swaziland where infections are nearly halved since 2011 (PEPFAR 2017). Efforts at "decentralization" in Mozambique continue to be closely chaperoned by outside agencies, including Vanderbilt, which undertakes management mentoring and other pilot projects in Zambézia Province (Edwards et al. 2015). That activist demands have become so mainstream symbolizes success, but where do they go from here?

REFERENCES

Abrahamsen, Rita. 2004. "The Power of Partnerships in Global Governance." *Third World Quarterly* 25 (8): 1453–1467.

Abrahamsson, Hans. 1997. *Seizing the Opportunity: Power and Powerlessness in a Changing World Order: The Case of Mozambique*. Gothenburg, Sweden: Dept. of Peace and Development Research, Gothenburg University.

Abt Associates Inc. 2012. *Health Systems 20/20: Final Project Report*. Bethesda, Md.: USAID.

Adams, Vincanne. 2016. Introduction to *Metrics: What Counts in Global Health*, 1. Reprint, Durham, N.C.: Duke University Press.

Afzal, Aasim, Mina Benjamin, Kyle L. Gummelt, et al. 2015. "Ascending Paralysis Associated with HIV Infection." *Proceedings (Baylor University. Medical Center)* 28 (1): 25–28.

Agência de Notícias de Resposta ao SIDA. 2009. "CNCS Passa Por Mudanças." *Abraço VIH-notícias* (blog). October 10, 2009. https://vihsidanoticias.wordpress.com/2009/10/10/mocambique-cncs-passa-por-mudancas/.

Alcano, Matteo Carlo. 2009. "Living and Working in Spite of Antiretroviral Therapies: Strength in Chronicity." *Anthropology and Medicine* 16 (2): 119–130.

Alden, Chris, and Sérgio Chichava, eds. 2014. *China and Mozambique: From Comrades to Capitalists*. Auckland Park, South Africa: Jacana Media.

Ancelovici, Marcos. 2015. "Crisis and Contention in Europe: A Political Process Account of Anti-austerity Protests." In *Europe's Prolonged Crisis*, 189–209. London, U.K.: Palgrave Macmillan.

Archer, Margaret S. 1995. *Realist Social Theory: The Morphogenetic Approach*. Cambridge: Cambridge University Press.

Atun, Rifat, Thyra de Jongh, Federica Secci, et al. 2010. "A Systematic Review of the Evidence on Integration of Targeted Health Interventions into Health Systems." *Health Policy and Planning* 25 (1): 1–14.

Auld, Andrew F., Ray W. Shiraishi, Aleny Couto, et al. 2016. "A Decade of Antiretroviral Therapy Scale-Up in Mozambique: Evaluation of Outcome Trends and New Models of Service Delivery among More Than 300,000 Patients Enrolled during 2004–2013." *Journal of Acquired Immune Deficiency Syndromes* 73 (2): e11–22.

Bademli, Kerime, and Zekiye Çetinkaya Duman. 2014. "Effects of a Family-to-Family Support Program on the Mental Health and Coping Strategies of Caregivers of Adults with Mental Illness: A Randomized Controlled Study." *Archives of Psychiatric Nursing* 28 (6): 392–398.

Bähre, Erik. 2007. "Reluctant Solidarity: Death, Urban Poverty, and Neighbourly Assistance in Urban South Africa." *Ethnography* 8 (1): 33–59.

Barlett, John A., and John F. Shao. 2009. "Successes, Challenges, and Limitations of Current Antiretroviral Therapy in Low-Income and Middle-Income Countries." *Lancet Infectious Diseases* 9 (10): 637–649.

Bärnighausen, Till, Krisda Chaiyachati, Natsayi Chimbindi, et al. 2011. "Interventions to Increase Antiretroviral Adherence in Sub-Saharan Africa: A Systematic Review of Evaluation Studies." *Lancet Infectious Diseases* 11 (12): 942–951.

Bastos, Cristiana. 2002. *Ciência, Poder, Acção: As Respostas à Sida*. Lisboa, Portugal: Imprensa de Ciéncias Sociais.

———. 2007. "Medical Hybridisms and Social Boundaries: Aspects of Portuguese Colonialism in Africa and India in the Nineteenth Century." *Journal of Southern African Studies* 33 (4): 767–782.

Bedelu, Martha, Nathan Ford, Katherine Hilderbrand, et al. 2007. "Implementing Antiretroviral Therapy in Rural Communities: The Lusikisiki Model of Decentralized HIV/AIDS Care." *Journal of Infectious Diseases* 196 (S3): S464–468.

Bell, Morag, Eugene Palka, Christopher Thurber, et al. 1999. *Therapeutic Landscapes: The Dynamic between Place and Wellness*. Edited by Allison Williams. Lanham, Md.: University Press of America.

Bemelmans, Marielle, Thomas van den Akker, Nathan Ford, et al. 2010. "Providing Universal Access to Antiretroviral Therapy in Thyolo, Malawi through Task Shifting and Decentralization of HIV/AIDS Care." *Tropical Medicine & International Health* 15 (12): 1413–1420.

Benford, Robert D., and David A. Snow. 2000. "Framing Processes and Social Movements: An Overview and Assessment." *Annual Review of Sociology* 26:611–639.

Benton, Adia. 2015. *HIV Exceptionalism: Development through Disease in Sierra Leone*. Minneapolis: University of Minnesota Press.

Berger, Peter L. 1970. *A Rumor of Angels: Modern Society and the Rediscovery of the Supernatural*. Garden City, N.Y.: Anchor.

———. 1990. *The Sacred Canopy: Elements of a Sociological Theory of Religion*. Reprint, New York: Anchor.

Berger, Peter L., and Thomas Luckmann. 1967. *The Social Construction of Reality: A Treatise in the Sociology of Knowledge*. New York: Anchor.

Berliner, Lauren S., and Nora J. Kenworthy. 2017. "Producing a Worthy Illness: Personal Crowdfunding amidst Financial Crisis." *Social Science & Medicine* 187:233–242.

Beyrer, Chris, Andrea L. Wirtz, Damian Walker, et al. 2011. *The Global HIV Epidemics among Men Who Have Sex with Men*. Washington, D.C.: The World Bank.

Biehl, João. 2006. "Pharmaceutical Governance." In *Global Pharmaceuticals: Ethics, Markets, Practices*, edited by Adriana Petryna, Andrew Lakoff, and Arthur Kleinman, 206–239. Durham, N.C.: Duke University Press.

Biehl, João, and Torben Eskerod. 2009. *Will to Live: AIDS Therapies and the Politics of Survival*. Princeton, N.J.: Princeton University Press.

Binagwaho, Agnes, and Niloo Ratnayake. 2009. "The Role of Social Capital in Successful Adherence to Antiretroviral Therapy in Africa." *PLOS Med* 6 (1): e18.

Bion, Wilfred. 1991. *Experiences in Groups: And Other Papers*. London: Routledge.

Birn, Anne-Emanuelle. 2009. "The Stages of International (Global) Health: Histories of Success or Successes of History?" *Global Public Health* 4 (1): 50–68.

Biruk, Crystal. 2012. "Seeing Like a Research Project: Producing 'High-Quality Data' in AIDS Research in Malawi." *Medical Anthropology* 31 (4): 347–366.

Bonate, Liazzat J. K. 2015. "The Advent and Schisms of Sufi Orders in Mozambique, 1896–1964." *Islam and Christian–Muslim Relations* 26 (4): 483–501.

Bor, Jacob, Shahira Ahmed, Matthew P. Fox, et al. 2017. "Effect of Eliminating CD4-Count Thresholds on HIV Treatment Initiation in South Africa: An Empirical Modeling Study." *PLOS ONE* 12 (6): e0178249.

Brinkhof, Martin W. G., Ben D. Spycher, Constantin Yiannoutsos, et al. 2010. "Adjusting Mortality for Loss to Follow-Up: Analysis of Five ART Programmes in Sub-Saharan Africa." *PLOS ONE* 5 (11): e14149.

Britten, Nicky. 1996. "Lay Views of Drugs and Medicines: Orthodox and Unorthodox Accounts." In *Modern Medicine: Lay Perspectives and Experiences*, edited by Simon J. Williams, 48–73. London: Routledge.

Brooks, Andrew. 2017. "Was Africa Rising? Narratives of Development Success and Failure among the Mozambican Middle Class." *Territory, Politics, Governance*: 1–21.

Brown, Julian. 2015. *South Africa's Insurgent Citizens: On Dissent and the Possibility of Politics*. London: Zed Books.

Brummelhuis, Han ten, and Gilbert Herdt, eds. 2004. *Culture and Sexual Risk*. New York: Routledge.

Bucagu, Maurice, Jean M. Kagubare, Paulin Basinga, et al. 2012. "Impact of Health Systems Strengthening on Coverage of Maternal Health Services in Rwanda, 2000–2010: A Systematic Review." *Reproductive Health Matters* 20 (39): 50–61.

Burchell, Graham. 1993. "Liberal Government and Techniques of the Self." *Economy and Society* 22 (3): 267–282.

Burnett, Alan, and Graham Moon. 1983. "Community Opposition to Hostels for Single Homeless Men." *Area* 15 (2): 161–166.

Cabassi, Julia, and David Wilson. 2005. "Renewing Our Voice: Code of Good Practice for NGOs Responding to HIV/AIDS." The 3 by 5 Initiative. http://www.who.int/3by5/partners/NGOcode/en/.

Caldwell, Christopher. 2017. "American Carnage." First Things. https://www.firstthings.com/article/2017/04/american-carnage.

Carter, Erika, and Simon Watney. 1997. *Taking Liberties: AIDS and Cultural Politics*. London: Serpent's Tail.

Casswell, Sally, and Anna Maxwell. 2005. "Regulation of Alcohol Marketing: A Global View." *Journal of Public Health Policy* 26 (3): 343–358.

Chabal, Patrick, David Birmingham, Joshua Forrest, et al. 2002. *A History of Postcolonial Lusophone Africa*. Bloomington, Ind.: Indiana University Press.

Chambré, Susan M. 2006. *Fighting for Our Lives: New York's AIDS Community and the Politics of Disease*. New Brunswick, NJ: Rutgers University Press.

Chan, Jennifer. 2015. *Politics in the Corridor of Dying: AIDS Activism and Global Health Governance*. Baltimore, Md.: Johns Hopkins University Press.

Chase, Sabrina. 2011. *Surviving HIV/AIDS in the Inner City: How Resourceful Latinas Beat the Odds*. New Brunswick, N.J.: Rutgers University Press.

Chewning, Lisa V., and Beth Montemurro. 2016. "The Structure of Support: Mapping Network Evolution in an Online Support Group." *Computers in Human Behavior* 64:355–365.

Cohen, Rachel, Sharonann Lynch, Helen Bygrave, et al. 2009. "Antiretroviral Treatment Outcomes from a Nurse-Driven, Community-Supported HIV/AIDS Treatment Programme in Rural Lesotho: Observational Cohort Assessment at Two Years." *Journal of the International AIDS Society* 12 (1): 23.

Colvin, Christopher J. 2014. "Evidence and AIDS Activism: HIV Scale-Up and the Contemporary Politics of Knowledge in Global Public Health." *Global Public Health* 9 (1/2): 57–72.

Conrad, Peter. 1985. "The Meaning of Medications: Another Look at Compliance." *Social Science & Medicine* 20 (1): 29–37.

Crane, Johanna Tayloe. 2013. *Scrambling for Africa: AIDS, Expertise, and the Rise of American Global Health Science*. Ithaca, N.Y.: Cornell University Press.

Cunguara, Benedito, and Joseph Hanlon. 2012. "Whose Wealth Is It Anyway? Mozambique's Outstanding Economic Growth with Worsening Rural Poverty." *Development and Change* 43 (3): 623–647.

Curtis, Sarah, Wil Gesler, Kathy Fabian, et al. 2007. "Therapeutic Landscapes in Hospital Design: A Qualitative Assessment by Staff and Service Users of the Design of a New Mental Health Inpatient Unit." *Environment and Planning C: Government and Policy* 25 (4): 591–610.

Daniel, Marguerite. 2014. "Iatrogenic Violence? Lived Experiences of Recipients of Aid That Targets Vulnerable Children in Makete, Tanzania." *Forum for Development Studies* 41 (3): 415–431.

Dear, Michael J., and Jennifer R. Wolch. 1987. *Landscapes of Despair: From Deinstitutionalization to Homelessness.* Princeton, N.J.: Princeton University Press.

Decroo, Tom, Isabella Panunzi, Carla das Dores, et al. 2009. "Lessons Learned during Down Referral of Antiretroviral Treatment in Tete, Mozambique." *Journal of the International AIDS Society* 12:6.

Decroo, Tom, Olivier Koole, Daniel Remartinez, et al. 2014. "Four-Year Retention and Risk Factors for Attrition among Members of Community ART Groups in Tete, Mozambique." *Tropical Medicine & International Health* 19 (5): 514–521.

Delisle, Vanessa C., Stephanie T. Gumuchian, Danielle B. Rice, et al. 2017. "Perceived Benefits and Factors That Influence the Ability to Establish and Maintain Patient Support Groups in Rare Diseases: A Scoping Review." *The Patient—Patient-Centered Outcomes Research* 10 (3): 283–293.

Denison, Julie A., Olivier Koole, Sharon Tsui, et al. 2015. "Incomplete Adherence among Treatment-Experienced Adults on Antiretroviral Therapy in Tanzania, Uganda and Zambia." *AIDS* 29 (3): 361–371.

DiMaggio, Paul J., and Walter W. Powell. 1983. "The Iron Cage Revisited: Institutional Isomorphism and Collective Rationality in Organizational Fields." *American Sociological Review* 48 (2): 147–160.

Donnelly, John. 2001. "Prevention Urged in AIDS Fight Natsios Says Fund Should Spend Less on HIV Treatment." *Boston Globe,* June 7, 2001.

DREAM. 2009. "Doentes de SIDA Acusam Ivo Garrido de Não Consultá-Los." *DREAM* (blog), August 10, 2009. http://dream.santegidio.org/2009/08/10/diario-de-noticias-mocambiquedoentes-de-sida-acusam-ivo-garrido-de-nao-consulta-los/.

Eade, John, and Michael Peter Smith. 2011. *Transnational Ties: Cities, Migrations, and Identities.* Piscataway, N.J.: Transaction Publishers.

Edwards, Laura J., Abú Moisés, Mathias Nzaramba, et al. 2015. "Implementation of a Health Management Mentoring Program: Year-1 Evaluation of Its Impact on Health System Strengthening in Zambézia Province, Mozambique." *International Journal of Health Policy and Management* 4 (6): 353–361.

Ekeh, Peter P. 1975. "Colonialism and the Two Publics in Africa: A Theoretical Statement." *Comparative Studies in Society and History* 17 (1): 91–112.

El-Sadr, Wafaa M., Miriam Rabkin, Rifat Atun, et al. 2011. "Bridging the Divide." *Journal of Acquired Immune Deficiency Syndromes* 57 (S2): S59–60.

Epstein, Steven. 1996. *Impure Science: AIDS, Activism, and the Politics of Knowledge.* Berkeley: University of California Press.

Evans, Alfred B., Laura A. Henry, and Lisa Sundstrom. 2016. *Russian Civil Society: A Critical Assessment.* Abingdon, U.K.: Routledge.

Farmer, Paul. 2006. *AIDS and Accusation: Haiti and the Geography of Blame.* Berkeley: University of California Press.

Fassin, Didier. 2007. *When Bodies Remember: Experiences and Politics of AIDS in South Africa.* Berkeley: University of California Press.

Fenio, Kenly Greer. 2009. "Between Bedrooms and Ballots: The Politics of HIV's 'Economy of Infection' in Mozambique." PhD diss., University of Florida.

———. 2011. "Tactics of Resistance and the Evolution of Identity from Subjects to Citizens: The AIDS Political Movement in Southern Africa." *International Studies Quarterly* 55 (3): 717–735.

Ferguson, James. 1994. *The Anti-politics Machine*. Minneapolis: University of Minnesota Press.

FHI 360. 2016. "Health Systems Strengthening." FHI 360. http://www.fhi360.org/expertise/health-systems-strengthening.

Foucault, Michel. 2010. *The Birth of Biopolitics: Lectures at the Collège de France, 1978–1979*. Reprint, New York: Picador.

France, David. 2016. *How to Survive a Plague: The Inside Story of How Citizens and Science Tamed AIDS*. New York: Knopf.

Frankl, Viktor E. 2006. *Man's Search for Meaning*. Boston: Beacon Press.

Friedman, Thomas L. 2005. *The World Is Flat: A Brief History of the Twenty-First Century*. New York: Farrar, Straus and Giroux.

Gamson, Josh. 1989. "Silence, Death, and the Invisible Enemy: AIDS Activism and Social Movement 'Newness.'" *Social Problems* 36 (4): 351–367.

Gergen, Jessica, Erik Josephson, Martha Coe, et al. 2017. "Quality of Care in Performance-Based Financing: How It Is Incorporated in 32 Programs Across 28 Countries." *Global Health, Science and Practice* 5 (1): 90–107.

Gesler, W. M. 1992. "Therapeutic Landscapes: Medical Issues in Light of the New Cultural Geography." *Social Science & Medicine* 34 (7): 735–746.

Gisselquist, Rachel M., Helena Pérez Niño, and Philippe Le Billon. 2014. "Foreign Aid, Resource Rents, and State Fragility in Mozambique and Angola." *ANNALS of the American Academy of Political and Social Science* 656 (1): 79–96.

Glasser, Irene. 2010. *More Than Bread: Ethnography of a Soup Kitchen*. Tuscaloosa: University Alabama Press.

Goffman, Erving. 1986. *Stigma: Notes on the Management of Spoiled Identity*. Reissue, New York: Touchstone.

Grebe, Eduard. 2011. "The Treatment Action Campaign's Struggle for AIDS Treatment in South Africa: Coalition-Building through Networks." *Journal of Southern African Studies* 37 (4): 849–868.

Green, Edward C., and Allison Herling Ruark. 2011. *AIDS, Behavior, and Culture: Understanding Evidence-Based Prevention*. Walnut Creek, Calif.: Routledge.

Grépin, Karen A. 2011. "Leveraging HIV Programs to Deliver an Integrated Package of Health Services: Some Words of Caution." *Journal of Acquired Immune Deficiency Syndromes* 57 (S2): S77–79.

Groh, Kate, Carolyn M. Audet, Alberto Baptista, et al. 2011. "Barriers to Antiretroviral Therapy Adherence in Rural Mozambique." *BMC Public Health* 11:650.

Hacking, Ian. 2000. *The Social Construction of What?* Cambridge, Mass.: Harvard University Press.

Hafner, Tamara, and Jeremy Shiffman. 2013. "The Emergence of Global Attention to Health Systems Strengthening." *Health Policy and Planning* 28 (1): 41–50.

Hanlon, Joseph. 2004. "Do Donors Promote Corruption?: The Case of Mozambique." *Third World Quarterly* 25 (4): 747–763.

Hardon, Anita, and Eileen Moyer. 2014. "Anthropology of AIDS: Modes of Engagement." *Medical Anthropology* 33 (4): 255–262.

Harman, Sophie. 2007. "The World Bank: Failing the Multi-country AIDS Program, Failing HIV/AIDS." *Global Governance* 13 (4): 485–492.

Harries, Anthony D., Rony Zachariah, Stephen D. Lawn, et al. 2010. "Strategies to Improve Patient Retention on Antiretroviral Therapy in Sub-Saharan Africa." *Tropical Medicine & International Health* 15 (S1): 70–75.

Harris, Marvin. 1960. *Portugal's African "Wards"—A First-Hand Report on Labor and Education in Mocambique.* New York: American Committee on Africa.

Harvey, David. 1991. *The Condition of Postmodernity: An Enquiry into the Origins of Cultural Change.* Cambridge, Mass.: Wiley-Blackwell.

Hayden, Patrick. 2012. "The Human Right to Health and the Struggle for Recognition." *Review of International Studies* 38 (3): 569–588.

Heath, Katherine V., Joel Singer, Michael V. O'Shaughnessy, Julio S. G. Montaner, and Robert S. Hogg. 2002. "Intentional Nonadherence Due to Adverse Symptoms Associated with Antiretroviral Therapy." *Journal of Acquired Immune Deficiency Syndromes* 31 (2): 211–217.

Hendershot, Christian S., Susan A. Stoner, David W. Pantalone, and Jane M. Simoni. 2009. "Alcohol Use and Antiretroviral Adherence: Review and Meta-analysis." *Journal of Acquired Immune Deficiency Syndromes* 52 (2): 180–202.

Hill, Geoff. 2016. "There's a Crisis in Our Oceans, Illegal Fishing Dwarfs Ivory and Rhino Horn Poaching." *Mail and Guardian.* July 19, 2016. https://mg.co.za/article/2016-07-18-theres-a-crisis-in-our-oceans-illegal-fishing-dwarfs-ivory-and-rhino-horn-poaching/.

Hirsch, Jennifer S., Holly Wardlow, Daniel Jordan Smith, et al. 2010. *The Secret: Love, Marriage, and HIV.* Nashville: Vanderbilt University Press.

Ho, Karen. 2009. *Liquidated: An Ethnography of Wall Street.* Durham, N.C.: Duke University Press.

Høg, Erling. 2006. "Human Rights and Access to AIDS Treatment in Mozambique." *African Journal of AIDS Research* 5 (1): 49–60.

Hollen, Cecilia Van. 2013. *Birth in the Age of AIDS: Women, Reproduction, and HIV/AIDS in India.* Palo Alto, Calif.: Stanford University Press.

Hu, Amanda. 2017. "Reflections: The Value of Patient Support Groups." *Otolaryngology—Head and Neck Surgery* 156 (4): 587–588.

Huber, Peter. 2007. "The Coming Plague." *Wall Street Journal,* April 10, 2007.

Huis In 't Veld, Diana, Linda Skaal, Karl Peltzer, et al. 2012. "The Efficacy of a Brief Intervention to Reduce Alcohol Misuse in Patients with HIV in South Africa: Study Protocol for a Randomized Controlled Trial." *Trials* 13:190.

Hunter, Mark. 2010. *Love in the Time of AIDS: Inequality, Gender, and Rights in South Africa.* Bloomington: Indiana University Press.

Igreja, Victor. 2008. "Memories as Weapons: The Politics of Peace and Silence in Post–Civil War Mozambique." *Journal of Southern African Studies* 34 (3): 539–556.

IHME. 2015. *Financing Global Health 2014: Shifts in Funding as the MDG Era Closes.* Seattle, Wash.: IHME. http://www.healthdata.org/sites/default/files/files/policy_report/2015/FGH2014/IHME_FGH_2014_Brief.pdf.

Iliffe, John. 2006. *The African AIDS Epidemic: A History.* Athens: Ohio University Press.

Illich, Ivan. 1982. *Medical Nemesis: The Expropriation of Health.* New York: Pantheon.

IMF. 2014. *Mozambique Rising: Building a New Tomorrow.* Washington, D.C.: International Monetary Fund, Publication Services.

Imrie, Rob. 2005. *Accessible Housing: Quality, Disability and Design.* London: Routledge.

Ingram, Alan. 2010. "Biosecurity and the International Response to HIV/AIDS: Governmentality, Globalisation and Security." *Area* 42 (3): 293–301.

INS. 2010. *Inquérito Nacional de Prevalência, Riscos Comportamentais e Informação Sobre o HIV e SIDA Em Moçambique 2009*. Calverton, Md.: ICF Macro.

―――. 2015. *Inquérito de Indicadores de Imunização, Malária e HIV/SIDA Em Moçambique 2015 (IMASIDA)*. Rockville, Md.: ICF Internacional.

IRIN PlusNews. 2009a. "Fim de Hospitais-Dia Traz Estigma e Mau Atendimento." IRIN. http://www.irinnews.org/printreport.aspx?reportid=82664.

―――. 2009b. "Liga Contra Discriminação Volta a Promover Protestos." IRIN. http://www.irinnews.org/report/86075/mo%C3%87ambique-liga-contra-discrimina%C3%A7%C3%A3o-volta-a-promover-protestos.

―――. 2009c. "MOÇAMBIQUE: Sociedade Civil Cria Observatório Para Monitorar Qualidade No Atendimento." IRIN. http://www.irinnews.org/printreport.aspx?reportid=86248.

Isaacman, Allen F., and Barbara Isaacman. 1983. *Mozambique: From Colonialism to Revolution, 1900–1982*. Boulder, Colo.: Westview Press.

Janovicek, Nancy. 2007. *No Place to Go: Local Histories of the Battered Women's Shelter Movement*. Vancouver, British Columbia: University of Washington Press.

Jasper, James M. 2014. *Protest: A Cultural Introduction to Social Movements*. Cambridge, Mass.: Polity.

Jobarteh, Kebba, Ray W. Shiraishi, Inacio Malimane, et al. 2016. "Community ART Support Groups in Mozambique: The Potential of Patients as Partners in Care." *PLOS ONE* 11 (12): e0166444.

Jones, Cleve. 2016. *When We Rise: My Life in the Movement*. New York: Hachette Books.

Jones, Edgar. 2006. "Historical Approaches to Post-combat Disorders." *Philosophical Transactions: Biological Sciences* 361 (1468): 533–542.

Kalichman, Seth C., Tamar Grebler, Christina M. Amaral, et al. 2013. "Intentional Nonadherence to Medications among HIV Positive Alcohol Drinkers: Prospective Study of Interactive Toxicity Beliefs." *Journal of General Internal Medicine* 28 (3): 399–405.

Kalipeni, Ezekiel, Susan Craddock, Joseph R. Oppong, et al., eds. 2003. *HIV and AIDS in Africa: Beyond Epidemiology*. Malden, Mass.: Wiley-Blackwell.

Kalofonos, Ippolytus. 2008. "'All I Eat Is ARVS': Living with HIV/AIDS at the Dawn of the Treatment Era in Central Mozambique." PhD diss., University of California, San Francisco.

―――. 2010. "'All I Eat Is ARVs': The Paradox of AIDS Treatment Interventions in Central Mozambique." *Medical Anthropology Quarterly* 24 (3): 363–380.

―――. 2014. "'All They Do Is Pray': Community Labour and the Narrowing of 'Care' during Mozambique's HIV Scale-Up." *Global Public Health* 9 (1/2): 7–24.

Kapp, Clare. 2007. "XDR Tuberculosis Spreads across South Africa." *Lancet* 369 (9563): 729.

Kearns, R. A., and D. C. Collins. 2000. "New Zealand Children's Health Camps: Therapeutic Landscapes Meet the Contract State." *Social Science & Medicine* 51 (7): 1047–1059.

Kelsall, Tim. 2002. "Shop Windows and Smoke-Filled Rooms: Governance and the Re-politicisation of Tanzania." *Journal of Modern African Studies* 40 (4): 597–619.

Kenworthy, Nora J. 2014. "Participation, Decentralisation and Déjà Vu: Remaking Democracy in Response to AIDS?" *Global Public Health* 9 (1/2): 25–42.

Kingod, Natasja, Bryan Cleal, Ayo Wahlberg, et al. 2017. "Online Peer-to-Peer Communities in the Daily Lives of People with Chronic Illness: A Qualitative Systematic Review." *Qualitative Health Research* 27 (1): 89–99.

Koenig, Serena P., Fernet Léandre, and Paul E. Farmer. 2004. "Scaling-Up HIV Treatment Programmes in Resource-Limited Settings: The Rural Haiti Experience." *AIDS* 18 (S3): S21–25.

Kotanyi, Sophie, and Brigitte Krings-Ney. 2009. "Introduction of Culturally Sensitive HIV Prevention in the Context of Female Initiation Rites: An Applied Anthropological Approach in Mozambique." *African Journal of AIDS Research* 8 (4): 491–502.

Kraemer, Sebastian. 2010. "'Great Men' Need Not Apply." *BMJ: British Medical Journal* 340 (7759): 1263–1264.

Kranzer, Katharina, and Nathan Ford. 2011. "Unstructured Treatment Interruption of Antiretroviral Therapy in Clinical Practice: A Systematic Review." *Tropical Medicine & International Health* 16 (10): 1297–1313.

Kristofferson, Kirk, Katherine White, and John Peloza. 2014. "The Nature of Slacktivism: How the Social Observability of an Initial Act of Token Support Affects Subsequent Prosocial Action." *Journal of Consumer Research* 40 (6): 1149–1166.

Kula. 2008. *Análise Da Situação Do HIV e SIDA e Acesso Ao TARV Em Moçambique*. Maputo, Mozambique: Kula: Estudos & Pesquisas Aplicadas.

Lambdin, Barrot H., Mark A. Micek, Kenneth Sherr, et al. 2013. "Integration of HIV Care and Treatment in Primary Health Care Centers and Patient Retention in Central Mozambique: A Retrospective Cohort Study." *Journal of Acquired Immune Deficiency Syndromes* 62 (5): e146–152.

Lapierre, Dominique. 1990. *Plus grand que l'amour*. Paris: Robert Laffont.

Lawn, Joy E., Jon Rohde, Susan Rifkin, et al. 2008. "Alma-Ata 30 Years On: Revolutionary, Relevant, and Time to Revitalise." *Lancet* 372 (9642): 917–927.

Leibing, Annette, and Lawrence Cohen. 2006. *Thinking about Dementia: Culture, Loss, and the Anthropology of Senility*. New Brunswick, N.J.: Rutgers University Press.

Lemke, Thomas. 2001. "'The Birth of Bio-politics': Michel Foucault's Lecture at the Collège de France on Neo-liberal Governmentality." *Economy and Society* 30 (2): 190–207.

Livingston, Jonathan, Harriette Pipes McAdoo, and Catherine J. Mills. 2010. "Black Studies and Political Ideology as Predictors of Self-Esteem: A Call for a New Direction." *Journal of Black Studies* 40 (4): 726–744.

Loewenson, Rene, and David McCoy. 2004. "Access to Antiretroviral Treatment in Africa." *BMJ: British Medical Journal* 328(7434): 241–242.

Long, Lawrence, Alana Brennan, Matthew P. Fox, et al. 2011. "Treatment Outcomes and Cost-Effectiveness of Shifting Management of Stable ART Patients to Nurses in South Africa: An Observational Cohort." *PLOS Med* 8 (7): e1001055.

Lumiere Action. 2015. "Lumière Action." Plateforme ELSA. http://www.plateforme-elsa.org/structure/lumiere-action/.

Luque-Fernandez, Miguel Angel, Gilles Van Cutsem, Eric Goemaere, et al. 2013. "Effectiveness of Patient Adherence Groups as a Model of Care for Stable Patients on Antiretroviral Therapy in Khayelitsha, Cape Town, South Africa." *PLOS ONE* 8 (2): e56088.

MacIntyre, Alasdair C. 1999. *The MacIntyre Reader*. Edited by Kelvin Knight. Notre Dame, Ind.: University of Notre Dame Press.

Mafeje, Archie. 1976. "The Problem of Anthropology in Historical Perspective: An Inquiry into the Growth of the Social Sciences." *Canadian Journal of African Studies / Revue Canadienne Des Études Africaines* 10 (2): 307–333.

Marcis, Frédéric Le. 2012. "Struggling with AIDS in South Africa: The Space of the Everyday as a Field of Recognition." *Medical Anthropology Quarterly* 26 (4): 486–502.

Marcis, Frederic Le, and Judith Inggs. 2004. "The Suffering Body of the City." *Public Culture* 16 (3): 453–477.

Marsland, Rebecca. 2012. "(Bio)Sociality and HIV in Tanzania: Finding a Living to Support a Life." *Medical Anthropology Quarterly* 26 (4): 470–485.

Martinez, Francisco Lerma. 1989. *O Povo Macua e a Sua Cultura*. Lisboa, Portugal: Ministério da Educação, Instituto de Investigação Científica Tropical.

Matsinhe, Cristiano. 2008. *Tabula Rasa: DinâMica Da Resposta Moçambicana Ao HIV/SIDA*. Maputo, Mozambique: Kula.

Mattes, Dominik. 2014. "Caught in Transition: The Struggle to Live a 'Normal' Life with HIV in Tanzania." *Medical Anthropology* 33 (4): 270–287.

Mbuba, Caroline K., Anthony K. Ngugi, Greg Fegan, et al. 2012. "Risk Factors Associated with the Epilepsy Treatment Gap in Kilifi, Kenya: A Cross-Sectional Study." *Lancet Neurology* 11 (8): 688–696.

McGrath, Janet W., Margaret S. Winchester, David Kaawa-Mafigiri, et al. 2014. "Challenging the Paradigm: Anthropological Perspectives on HIV as a Chronic Disease." *Medical Anthropology* 33 (4): 303–317.

McLean, Athena. 2007. "The Therapeutic Landscape of Dementia Care: Contours of Intersubjective Spaces for Sustaining the Person." In *Therapeutic Landscapes: The Dynamic between Place and Wellness*, Edited by Allison Williams, Morag Bell, Christopher Thurber, et al. 315–332. Lanham, Md.: University Press of America.

Mercer, Mary Anne, Susan M. Thompson, and Rui Maria de Araujo. 2014. "The Role of International NGOs in Health Systems Strengthening: The Case of Timor-Leste." *International Journal of Health Services: Planning, Administration, Evaluation* 44 (2): 323–335.

Miller, Peter, and Nikolas Rose. 1994. "On Therapeutic Authority: Psychoanalytical Expertise under Advanced Liberalism." *History of the Human Sciences* 7 (3): 29–64.

Millikan, Ruth Garrett. 1987. *Language, Thought, and Other Biological Categories: New Foundations for Realism*. Reprint, Cambridge, Mass.: The MIT Press.

Mills, Edward J., Jean B. Nachega, Iain Buchan, et al. 2006. "Adherence to Antiretroviral Therapy in Sub-Saharan Africa and North America: A Meta-analysis." *JAMA* 296 (6): 679–690.

MISAU. 2004. *Hospitais de Dia e Cuidados Ambulatórios Para Pessoas Vivendo Com HIV/SIDA: Guião Para a Organização e Gestão. 20 Rascunho*. República de Moçambique: MISAU.

———. 2015. *National Program on HIV, AIDS, STIs 2014 Annual Report*. Maputo, Mozambique: Instituto Nacional de Saúde.

———. 2016. *Relatório Anual Das Actividades Relacionadas Ao HIV/SIDA*. Maputo, Mozambique: Serviço Nacional de Saúde.

———. 2017a. *National Program on HIV, AIDS, STIs 2016 Annual Report*. Maputo, Mozambique: Instituto Nacional de Saúde.

———. 2017b. *Relatorio de Indicadores Basicos de HIV*. Maputo, Mozambique: ICF Internacional.

Moyer, Eileen, and Anita Hardon. 2014. "A Disease Unlike Any Other? Why HIV Remains Exceptional in the Age of Treatment." *Medical Anthropology* 33 (4): 263–269.

Muhumuza, W. 2008. "Pitfalls of Decentralization Reforms in Transitional Societies: The Case of Uganda." *Africa Development* 33 (4): 59–81.

Munslow, Barry, ed. 1986. *Africa: Problems in the Transition to Socialism*. Atlantic Highlands, N.J.: Zed Books.

Mussa, Abdul H., James Pfeiffer, Stephen S. Gloyd, et al. 2013. "Vertical Funding, Nongovernmental Organizations, and Health System Strengthening: Perspectives of Public Sector Health Workers in Mozambique." *Human Resources for Health* 11:26.

Mutiua, Chapane. 2014. "Ajami Literacy, Class, and Portuguese Pre-colonial Administration in Northern Mozambique." PhD thesis, University of Cape Town. https://open.uct.ac.za/handle/11427/13183.

Nachega, Jean B., Michael Hislop, David W. Dowdy, et al. 2006. "Adherence to Highly Active Antiretroviral Therapy Assessed by Pharmacy Claims Predicts Survival in HIV-Infected South African Adults." *Journal of Acquired Immune Deficiency Syndromes* 43 (1): 78–84.

Naoi, Riyo. 2017. "Everyday Activities of Support Groups for HIV-Positive People in Northern Thailand." *Japanese Journal of Southeast Asian Studies* 54 (2): 182–204.

Nattrass, Nicoli. 2007. *Mortal Combat: AIDS Denialism and the Struggle for Antiretrovirals in South Africa.* Scottsville, South Africa: University Of KwaZulu-Natal Press.

Needle, Richard H., Susan L. Coyle, Jacques Normand, et al. 1998. "HIV Prevention with Drug-Using Populations: Current Status and Future Prospects: Introduction and Overview." *Public Health Reports* 113:4–18.

Newell, K. W. 1988. "Selective Primary Health Care: The Counter Revolution." *Social Science & Medicine* 26 (9): 903–906.

Newitt, M. D. D. 1972a. "The Early History of the Sultanate of Angoche." *Journal of African History* 13 (3): 397–406.

——. 1972b. "Angoche, the Slave Trade and the Portuguese c. 1844–1910." *Journal of African History* 13 (4): 659–672.

Nguyen, Vinh-Kim. 2007. "Antiretroviral Globalism, Biopolitics, and Therapeutic Citizenship." In *Global Assemblages*, edited by Aihwa Ong and Stephen J. Collier, 124–144. Hoboken, N.J.: Blackwell.

——. 2010. *The Republic of Therapy: Triage and Sovereignty in West Africa's Time of AIDS.* Durham, N.C.: Duke University Press.

Nguyen, Vinh-Kim, Cyriaque Yapo Ako, Pascal Niamba, et al. 2007. "Adherence as Therapeutic Citizenship: Impact of the History of Access to Antiretroviral Drugs on Adherence to Treatment." *AIDS* 21 (S5): S31–35.

Nicolson, Greg. 2014. "TAC: Funding, Accountability and the Dire Consequences of Closure." *Daily Maverick*, October 3, 2014.

Niehaus, Isak. 2014. "Treatment Literacy, Therapeutic Efficacy, and Antiretroviral Drugs: Notes from Bushbuckridge, South Africa." *Medical Anthropology* 33 (4): 351–366.

Nietzsche, Friedrich. 1989. *Beyond Good and Evil: Prelude to a Philosophy of the Future.* Translated by Walter Kaufmann. New York: Vintage.

Norton, Wynne E., K. Rivet Amico, William A. Fisher, et al. 2010. "Information-Motivation-Behavioral Skills Barriers Associated with Intentional versus Unintentional ARV Nonadherence Behavior among HIV+ Patients in Clinical Care." *AIDS Care* 22 (8): 979–987.

Nuwer, Deanne Stephens. 2009. *Plague among the Magnolias: The 1878 Yellow Fever Epidemic in Mississippi.* Tuscaloosa: University Alabama Press.

Ogundeji, Yewande Kofoworola, Cath Jackson, Trevor Sheldon, et al. 2016. "Pay for Performance in Nigeria: The Influence of Context and Implementation on Results." *Health Policy and Planning* 31 (8): 955–963.

O'Laughlin, Bridget. 2009. "Rural Social Security and the Limits of 'Associativismo' in Southern Mozambique." In II Conferencia de Instituto de Estudos Sociais e Económicos: *Dinamicas Da Pobreza e Padrões de Acumulação Económica Em Moçambique*, Maputo, Moçambique, 2009, 1–32. Maputo, Mozambique: IESE.

Olsen, Bent Steenberg. 2013. "Structures of Stigma: Diagonal AIDS Care and Treatment Abandonment in Mozambique." PhD diss., Roskilde University.

Oransky, Ivan. 2003. "African Patients Adhere Well to Anti-HIV Regimens." *Lancet* 362 (9387): 882.

Organization of African Unity. 1981. "African [Banjul] Charter on Human and Peoples' Rights." University of Minnesota Human Rights Library. http://www1.umn.edu/humanrts/instree/z1afchar.htm.

Owczarzak, Jill. 2010. "Activism, NGOs, and HIV Prevention in Postsocialist Poland: The Role of 'Anti-politics.'" *Human Organization* 69 (2): 200–211.

Parker, Richard, and Anke A. Ehrhardt. 2001. "Through an Ethnographic Lens: Ethnographic Methods, Comparative Analysis, and HIV/AIDS Research." *AIDS and Behavior* 5 (2): 105–114.

Parr, Hester, and Joyce Davidson. 2009. "Mental and Emotional Health." In *A Companion to Health and Medical Geography*, edited by Tim Brown, Sara McLafferty, and Graham Moon, 258–277. Malden, Mass.: Wiley-Blackwell.

Parry, Charles Dh, Neo K. Morojele, Bronwyn J. Myers, et al. 2014. "Efficacy of an Alcohol-Focused Intervention for Improving Adherence to Antiretroviral Therapy (ART) and HIV Treatment Outcomes—a Randomised Controlled Trial Protocol." *BMC Infectious Diseases* 14:500.

Patterson, Amy S. 2016. "Engaging Therapeutic Citizenship and Clientship: Untangling the Reasons for Therapeutic Pacifism among People Living with HIV in Urban Zambia." *Global Public Health* 11 (9): 1121–1134.

Paul, Elisabeth, and Dimitri Renmans. 2017. "Performance-Based Financing in the Heath Sector in Low- and Middle-Income Countries: Is There Anything Whereof It May Be Said, See, This Is New?" *The International Journal of Health Planning and Management.* https://onlinelibrary.wiley.com/doi/abs/10.1002/hpm.2409.

Paul, Elisabeth, Mohamed Lamine Dramé, Jean-Pierre Kashala, et al. 2017. Performance-Based Financing to Strengthen the Health System in Benin: Challenging the Mainstream Approach. International Journal of Health Policy and Management 0(0).

PBS Newshour. 2010. "High Costs of HIV Medication Cause 'Terrible Dilemma' in Mozambique." PBS Newshour. http://www.pbs.org/newshour.

PEPFAR. 2017. "Four African Countries Approaching Control of Their HIV Epidemics as U.S. Continues Its Commitment to PEPFAR." PEPFAR. https://www.pepfar.gov/press/releases/2017/272788.htm.

Petryna, Adriana. 2013. *Life Exposed: Biological Citizens after Chernobyl.* Princeton, N.J.: Princeton University Press.

Petryna, Adriana, Andrew Lakoff, and Arthur Kleinman, eds. 2006. *Global Pharmaceuticals: Ethics, Markets, Practices.* Durham, N.C.: Duke University Press.

Pfeiffer, James, and Rachel Chapman. 2010. "Anthropological Perspectives on Structural Adjustment and Public Health." *Annual Review of Anthropology* 39 (1): 149–165.

Pfeiffer, James, Pablo Montoya, Alberto J. Baptista, et al. 2010. "Integration of HIV/AIDS Services into African Primary Health Care: Lessons Learned for Health System Strengthening in Mozambique—a Case Study." *Journal of the International AIDS Society* 13 (1): 3.

Philbin, Morgan M. 2014. "'What I Got to Go Through': Normalization and HIV-Positive Adolescents." *Medical Anthropology* 33 (4): 288–302.

Piel, Jonathon, ed. 1988. "What We Know about AIDS." *Scientific American* 259 (4): 1–152.

Pitcher, Anne, Mary H. Moran, and Michael Johnston. 2009. "Rethinking Patrimonialism and Neopatrimonialism in Africa." *African Studies Review* 52 (1): 125–156.

Pitcher, M. Anne. 2008. *Transforming Mozambique: The Politics of Privatization, 1975–2000.* Cambridge: Cambridge University Press.

Plagerson, Sophie. 2005. "Attacking Social Exclusion: Combining Rehabilitative and Preventive Approaches to Leprosy in Bangladesh." *Development in Practice* 15 (5): 692–700.

Porta, Donatella della, and Mario Diani. 2006. *Social Movements: An Introduction*. 2nd ed. Malden, Mass.: Wiley-Blackwell.

Powers, Theodore. 2012. "Institutionalising Dissent: HIV/AIDS, the Post-Apartheid State and the Limits of Transnational Governance in South Africa." *Journal of Southern African Studies* 38 (3): 531–549.

Prince, Ruth. 2012. "HIV and the Moral Economy of Survival in an East African City." *Medical Anthropology Quarterly* 26 (4): 534–556.

Quinn, Ben. 2016. "Mozambique Debt Crisis Could Be First Sign of Global Financial Shockwave." *Guardian*, October 27, 2016. https://www.theguardian.com/global-development/2016/oct/27/mozambique-debt-crisis-first-sign-global-financial-shockwave.

Rabinow, Paul. 1996. "Artificiality and Enlightenment: From Sociobiology to Biosociality." In *Anthropologies of Modernity*, edited by Jonathan Xavier Inda, 179–193. Hoboken, N.J.: Blackwell.

Rabkin, Miriam, and Sania Nishtar. 2011. "Scaling Up Chronic Care Systems: Leveraging HIV Programs to Support Noncommunicable Disease Services." *Journal of Acquired Immune Deficiency Syndromes* 57 (S2): S87–90.

Rau, Bill. 2006. "The Politics of Civil Society in Confronting HIV / AIDS." *International Affairs* 82 (2): 285–295.

Ray, Amy L., and Steven R. Gold. 1996. "Gender Roles, Aggression, and Alcohol Use in Dating Relationships." *Journal of Sex Research* 33 (1): 47–55.

Reed, Joel Christian. 2005. "HIV/AIDS Workplace Interventions in South Africa and the United States." PhD diss., University of South Florida. http://scholarcommons.usf.edu/etd/831.

Renmans, Dimitri, Nathalie Holvoet, Christopher Garimoi Orach, et al. 2016. "Opening the 'Black Box' of Performance-Based Financing in Low- and Lower Middle-Income Countries: A Review of the Literature." *Health Policy and Planning* 31 (9): 1297–1309.

República de Moçambique. 2009. *Direitos e Deveres Da Pessoa Vivendo Com HIV e SIDA* 1 (10).

Roberts, Sandra. 2008. "Normative Functions of HIV/AIDS Support Groups." *South African Review of Sociology* 39 (1): 83–97.

Robins, Steven. 2004. "'Long Live Zackie, Long Live': AIDS Activism, Science and Citizenship after Apartheid." *Journal of Southern African Studies* 30 (3): 651–672.

———. 2006. "From 'Rights' to 'Ritual': AIDS Activism in South Africa." *American Anthropologist* 108 (2): 312–323.

———. 2010. *From Revolution to Rights in South Africa*. Reprint, Cape Town, South Africa: BOYE6.

Rose, Nikolas, and Carlos Novas. 2005. "Biological Citizenship." In *Global Assemblages*, edited by Aihwa Ong and Stephen J. Collier, 439–463. Hoboken, N.J.: Blackwell.

Rosen, Michael. 2012. *Dignity: Its History and Meaning*. Cambridge, Mass.: Harvard University Press.

Ross, Richard S. 2015. *Contagion in Prussia, 1831 the Cholera Epidemic and the Threat of the Polish Uprising*. Jefferson, N.C.: McFarland.

Roth, Benita. 2017. *The Life and Death of ACT UP/LA: Anti-AIDS Activism in Los Angeles from the 1980s to the 2000s*. New York: Cambridge University Press.

Rucht, Dieter. 2007. "The Spread of Protest Politics." In *The Oxford Handbook of Political Behavior*, edited by Russell Dalton and Hans-Dieter Klingemann. Oxford, U.K.: Oxford University Press.

Sabatier, Tade Aina, and Jon Tinker Renee. 1987. *Blaming Others: Racial and Ethnic Aspects of AIDS*. London: Panos.

Sangaramoorthy, Thurka, and Adia Benton. 2012. "Enumeration, Identity, and Health." *Medical Anthropology* 31 (4): 287–291.

Santos, Boaventura de Sousa. 2005. "Beyond Neoliberal Governance: The World Social Forum as Subaltern Cosmopolitan Politis and Legality." In *Law and Globalization from Below: Towards a Cosmopolitan Legality*, edited by Boaventura de Sousa Santos and César A. Rodríguez-Garavito, 29–63. Cambridge: Cambridge University Press.

Savana. 2008. "Garrido Denies Ordering Closure of Day Hospitals." Club of Mozambique. http://www.clubofmozambique.com/solutions1/sectionnews.php?id=11286&tipo=one.

Schafer, Jessica. 2001. "Guerrillas and Violence in the War in Mozambique: De-socialization or Re-socialization?" *African Affairs* 100 (399): 215–237.

Schneider, Helen, Duane Blaauw, Lucy Gilson, et al. 2006. "Health Systems and Access to Antiretroviral Drugs for HIV in Southern Africa: Service Delivery and Human Resources Challenges." *Reproductive Health Matters* 14 (27): 12–23.

Scott, J., Elizabeth A. McCallion, Tessa Frohe, et al. 2017. "Lifetime Alcoholics Anonymous Attendance as a Predictor of Spiritual Gains in the Relapse Replication and Extension Project (RREP)." *Psychology of Addictive Behaviors* 31 (1): 54–60.

Sekhri, Neelam. 2006. *From Funding to Action: Strengthening Healthcare Systems in Sub-Saharan Africa*. Cologny, Switzerland: Becton, Dickinson, and Company.

Serapião, Luís Benjamim. 2004. "The Catholic Church and Conflict Resolution in Mozambique's Post-colonial Conflict, 1977–1992." *Journal of Church and State* 46 (2): 365–387.

Shilts, Randy. 1987. *And the Band Played On: Politics, People, and the AIDS Epidemic*. New York: St. Martin's Press.

Shotwell, Alexis. 2016. *Against Purity: Living Ethically in Compromised Times*. Minneapolis: University of Minnesota Press.

Simoni, Jane M., Ann E. Kurth, Cynthia R. Pearson, et al. 2006. "Self-Report Measures of Antiretroviral Therapy Adherence: A Review with Recommendations for HIV Research and Clinical Management." *AIDS and Behavior* 10 (3): 227–245.

Singer, Merrill. 2005. *The Face of Social Suffering: Life History of a Street Drug Addict*. Long Grove, Ill: Waveland Press.

Singer, Merrill, Nicola Bulled, Bayla Ostrach, et al. 2017. "Syndemics and the Biosocial Conception of Health." *Lancet* 389 (10072): 941–950.

Smith, Alesha J., and Susan E. Tett. 2010. "Improving the Use of Benzodiazepines—Is It Possible? A Non-systematic Review of Interventions Tried in the Last 20 Years." *BMC Health Services Research* 10:321.

Smith, Raymond. 2013. "Can There Be a Fourth Great Wave of AIDS Activism?" *Huffington Post*, February 2, 2016. http://www.huffingtonpost.com/raymond-a-smith-phd/can-there-be-a-fourth-great-wave-of-aids-activism_b_4171233.html.

Smith, Raymond A., and Patricia D. Siplon. 2006. *Drugs into Bodies: Global AIDS Treatment Activism*. Westport, Conn.: Praeger.

Soeters, Robert, Peter Bob Peerenboom, Pacifique Mushagalusa, et al. 2011. "Performance-Based Financing Experiment Improved Health Care in the Democratic Republic of Congo." *Health Affairs* 30 (8): 1518–1527.

Sontag, Susan. 1989. *Aids and Its Metaphors*. 2nd ed. New York: New York Review of Books.

Spencer, Dale C., and Kevin Walby. 2013. "Neo-tribalism, Epistemic Cultures, and the Emotions of Scientific Knowledge Construction." *Emotion, Space and Society* 7:54–61.

Spisak, Cary, Lindsay Morgan, Rena Eichler, et al. 2016. "Results-Based Financing in Mozambique's Central Medical Store: A Review after 1 Year." *Global Health: Science and Practice* 4 (1): 165–177.

Steffen, Vibeke. 2005. *Managing Uncertainty: Ethnographic Studies of Illness, Risk and the Struggle for Control.* Copenhagen, Denmark: Museum Tusculanum Press.

Storeng, Katerini T. 2014. "The GAVI Alliance and the 'Gates Approach' to Health System Strengthening." *Global Public Health* 9 (8): 865–879.

Suarez, Ray. 2010. "Mozambique's Health Care Struggles Put Need for Basics Back in Focus." PBS NewsHour. http://www.pbs.org/newshour/rundown/mozambiques-health-system -a-maze-of-need/.

Sumich, Jason. 2013. "Tenuous Belonging: Citizenship and Democracy in Mozambique." *Social Analysis* 57 (2): 99–116.

Sundell, Knut, and Lars Wärngård. 2013. *How Do Government Agencies Use Evidence?* Stockholm, Sweden: National Board of Health and Welfare.

Susser, Ida. 2009. *AIDS, Sex, and Culture: Global Politics and Survival in Southern Africa.* Chichester, U.K.: Wiley-Blackwell.

Suthar, Amitabh B., Jason M. Nagata, Sabin Nsanzimana, et al. 2017. "Performance-Based Financing for Improving HIV/AIDS Service Delivery: A Systematic Review." *BMC Health Services Research* 17. http://www.ncbi.nlm.nih.gov/pmc/articles/PMC5210258.

Tarrow, Sidney. 2011. *Power in Movement: Social Movements and Contentious Politics.* 3rd ed. Cambridge, Mass.: Cambridge University Press.

Tarrow, Sidney, and Charles Tilly. 2009. "Contentious Politics and Social Movements." In *The Oxford Handbook of Comparative Politics,* edited by Carles Boix and Susan C. Stokes, 435–460. Oxford, U.K.: Oxford University Press.

't Hoen, Ellen. 2002. "TRIPS, Pharmaceutical Patents, and Access to Essential Medicines: A Long Way from Seattle to Doha." *Chicago Journal of International Law* 3 (1): 27–46.

Thörn, Håkan. 2016. "Politics of Responsibility: Governing Distant Populations through Civil Society in Mozambique, Rwanda and South Africa." *Third World Quarterly* 37 (8): 1505–1523.

Trostle, J. A. 1988. "Medical Compliance as an Ideology." *Social Science & Medicine* 27 (12): 1299–1308.

Tusalem, Rollin F. 2007. "A Boon or a Bane? The Role of Civil Society in Third- and Fourth-Wave Democracies." *International Political Science Review / Revue Internationale de Science Politique* 28 (3): 361–386.

UNAIDS. 2006. "Report on the Global AIDS Epidemic." UNAIDS. http://www.unaids.org.

———. 2012. "Treatment 2015." UNAIDS. http://www.unaids.org/sites/default/files/ media_asset/JC2484_treatment-2015_en_1.pdf.

———. 2013. "Access to Antiretroviral Therapy in Africa: Status on Report Progress towards the 2015 Targets." UNAIDS. http://www.unaids.org/en/resources/documents/2013/ 20131219_AccessARTAfricaStatusReportProgresstowards2015Targets.

———. 2016a. "Resposta Global à SIDA, Relatório Do Progresso, Moçambique." WHO. http://www.who.int/hiv/pub/arv/global-aids-update-2016-pub/en/.

———. 2016b. "AIDS Data." UNAIDS. http://www.unaids.org/sites/default/files/media _asset/2016-AIDS-data_en.pdf.

———. 2017. "Global AIDS Update." UNAIDS. http://www.unaids.org.

UNDP. 2016. *Human Development Report—Mozambique.* Geneva, Switzerland: UNDP.

United Nations Office of the High Commissioner for Human Rights. 1966. "International Covenant on Economic, Social and Cultural Rights." United Nations Office of the High Commissioner for Human Rights. http://www.ohchr.org/EN/ProfessionalInterest/ Pages/CESCR.aspx.

U.S. Department of State. 2014. "Trafficking in Persons Report." U. S. Department of State. http://www.state.gov/j/tip/rls/tiprpt/countries/2014/226783.htm.

Vallée, Jean-Marc, dir. 2013. *Dallas Buyers Club*; Los Angeles: Focus Features.

Valverde, Mariana, and Kimberley White-Mair. 1999. "'One Day at a Time' and Other Slogans for Everyday Life: The Ethical Practices of Alcoholics Anonymous." *Sociology* 33 (2): 393–410.

Van Damme, Wim, and Guy Kegels. 2006. "Health System Strengthening and Scaling up Antiretroviral Therapy: The Need for Context-Specific Delivery Models: Comment on Schneider et Al." *Reproductive Health Matters* 14 (27): 24–26.

Verdade. 2009. "Hospitais Dia Não Tem Lugar No Ordenamento Nacional," *Verdade*, August 5, 2009. http://www.verdade.co.mz/saude-e-bem-estar/4269-hospitais-dia-nao-tem-lugar-no-ordenamento-nacional.

Vines, Alex. 1991. *Renamo: Terrorism in Mozambique*. Bloomington: Indiana University Press.

Wallace, R. 1990. "Urban Desertification, Public Health and Public Order: 'Planned Shrinkage,' Violent Death, Substance Abuse and AIDS in the Bronx." *Social Science & Medicine* 31 (7): 801–813.

Walsh, J. A., and K. S. Warren. 1979. "Selective Primary Health Care: An Interim Strategy for Disease Control in Developing Countries." *New England Journal of Medicine* 301 (18): 967–974.

Walton, David A., Paul E. Farmer, Wesler Lambert, et al. 2004. "Integrated HIV Prevention and Care Strengthens Primary Health Care: Lessons from Rural Haiti." *Journal of Public Health Policy* 25 (2): 137–158.

Wamba, Lucrecia Jose, and Tiwonge Towera Loga. 2008. "Southern African AIDS Trust (SAT) Commitment for a Coordinated Response to HIV and AIDS in Southern Africa: The Implementation of the 'Three Ones.'" *Canadian Journal of Public Health / Revue Canadienne de Sante'e Publique* 99:S11–S15.

Wardman, Anna. 1985. "The Co-operative Movement in Chokwe, Mozambique." *Journal of Southern African Studies* 11 (2): 295–304.

Ware, Norma C., John Idoko, Sylvia Kaaya, et al. 2009. "Explaining Adherence Success in Sub-Saharan Africa: An Ethnographic Study." *PLOS Med* 6 (1): e1000011.

Warren, Ashley E., Kaspar Wyss, George Shakarishvili, et al. 2013. "Global Health Initiative Investments and Health Systems Strengthening: A Content Analysis of Global Fund Investments." *Globalization & Health* 9 (1): 1–14.

West, Harry. 2008. "'Govern Yourselves': Democracy and Carnage in Northern Mozambique." In *Towards an Anthropology of Knowledge*, 97–121. Santa Fe, N.Mex.: School of Advanced Research.

West, Harry G. 2005. *Kupilikula: Governance and the Invisible Realm in Mozambique*. Chicago: University of Chicago Press.

WHO. 1948. "The Universal Declaration of Human Rights." WHO. http://www.un.org/en/documents/udhr/.

———. 2000. "The Kaya Kwanga Commitment." WHO. http://www.who.int/countries/moz/publications/kaya_kwanga/en/.

———. 2007. "Everybody's Business: Strengthening Health Systems to Improve Health Outcomes: WHO's Framework for Action." WHO. http://www.who.int/healthsystems/strategy/everybodys_business.pdf.

———. 2009. "Towards Universal Access: Scaling up Priority HIV/AIDS Interventions in the Health Sector." WHO. http://www.who.int/hiv/pub/2009progressreport/en/.

———. 2010. "Monitoring the Building Blocks of Health Systems: A Handbook of Indicators and Their Measurement Strategies." WHO. http://www.who.int/healthinfo/systems/monitoring/en/.

———. 2013. "Global Update on HIV Treatment 2013: Results, Impact and Opportunities." WHO. http://www.who.int/hiv/pub/progressreports/update2013/en/.

———. 2014. "Global Status Report on Alcohol and Health 2014." WHO. http://www.who.int/substance_abuse/publications/global_alcohol_report/en/.

Wilton, Robert, and Geoffrey Deverteuil. 2006. "Spaces of Sobriety/Sites of Power: Examining Social Model Alcohol Recovery Programs as Therapeutic Landscapes." *Social Science & Medicine* 63 (3): 649–661.

Winchester, Margaret S., Janet W. McGrath, David Kaawa-Mafigiri, et al. 2017. "Routines, Hope, and Antiretroviral Treatment among Men and Women in Uganda." *Medical Anthropology Quarterly* 31 (2): 237–256.

World Bank. 1992. "Governance and Development. 10650." The World Bank. http://documents.worldbank.org/curated/en/1992/04/440582/governance-development.

Zulu, W. 1993. "'Positive and Living' in Zambia." *AIDS Action* (21): 8.

INDEX

The letter *t* following a page number denotes a table.

UNAIDS, xvi, 17, 25; and AIDS advocacy,
34, 169; and Cysne, Mauricio, 131; and
decentralization, 125–127, 130, 134, 138;
and health systems strengthening, 141,
152; in Mozambique, 34, 168; and 3 by 5
initiative, 28

United States Agency for International Development, 25, 105, 168, 178n13

vergonha. See stigma

workshopocracy, 70–73
World AIDS Day, 136, 150

ABOUT THE AUTHOR

JOEL CHRISTIAN REED, PhD, MPH, is a medical anthropologist and epidemiologist from Lexington, Kentucky. He attended the University of Kentucky, the University of South Florida, and Michigan State University. He has worked with the Peace Corps, Doctors without Borders, and the Centers for Disease Control and Prevention and was a Fulbright Scholar. He currently works with the USAID-funded Demographic and Health Surveys Program at ICF, in Rockville, Maryland.

Printed in the United States
By Bookmasters